D1758284

Reference

022909

An Atlas of
RADIOLOGY OF
THE TRAUMATIZED
DOG & CAT

Joe P. Morgan, DVM, Vet. med. dr.
School of Veterinary Medicine
University of California
Davis
United States of America

Pim Wolvekamp, DVM, PhD
Faculty of Veterinary Medicine
University of Utrecht
The Netherlands

MANSON PUBLISHING/THE VETERINARY PRESS

Published 1994 by Manson Publishing/The Veterinary Press Ltd.,
73 Corringham Road, London NW11 7DL, UK
Copyright © 1994 Schlütersche Verlagsanstalt und
Druckerei GmbH & Co.,
Hans-Böckler-Allee 7, 30173 Hannover, Germany.
A CIP catalogue record for this publication is available from the British Library.
ISBN 1-874545-18-9

Copublished and distributed in North America by J. B. Lippincott Company,
227 East Washington Square, Philadelphia, PA 19106, 1994.
Library of Congress Cataloging-in-Publication Data applied for.
ISBN 0-397-51483-2

Printed by Schlütersche Verlagsanstalt und Druckerei GmbH & Co.

CONTENTS

PREFACE

The cornerstones of diagnostic radiology are good radiographic technique and accurate interpretation of the radiographs. This Atlas contains many useful technical hints for correct performance of the radiographic examination of traumatized animals. The radiographic characteristics of a diagnostic study are clearly defined. Most of the illustrations are non-contrast survey radiographs produced with an overhead tube and vertical X-ray beam. In addition, the application of simple contrast techniques for radiographic evaluation of abdominal trauma is discussed and the advantages of horizontally-beamed, cross-table radiography are suggested.

However, this atlas primarily emphasizes radiographic interpretation. For reasons of convenience, the text is divided into three major sections: thoracic trauma — abdominal trauma — musculoskeletal trauma. Within each section are discussions based on the characteristic radiographic changes of that area. For example, free peritoneal fluid in the abdominal cavity is discussed not only considering the resulting radiographic pattern but also the possible etiologies of the fluid. This is supported in the text by a table that conveniently lists the radiographic signs that can be used in the diagnosis of peritoneal fluid.

This Atlas is primarily directed towards the practicing veterinarian as an aid in his continual battle to diagnose and treat traumatized dogs and cats. The scope of this text is limited to these species. Most of the illustrated cases would be considered as emergency patients: some have life-threatening injuries, others traumatic injuries that simply need diagnosis and treatment. Many of the selected cases concern animals involved in automobile accidents, however, other types of traumatic injury are also presented.

Especially because of the inability of animals to communicate directly and the difficulty of performing a thorough and adequate physical examination with many traumatized animals, the immediate diagnosis of trauma cases is greatly assisted by the use of diagnostic radiology, often whole-body radiography. This dependence upon diagnostic radiology has made veterinary radiology an acknowledged specialty. However, in the middle of the night a specialist may not be available and most probably the veterinarian on call must make the first radiographic evaluation himself. At that moment, this Atlas will serve him. Students also can benefit from the Atlas since it describes the use of basic diagnostic radiology in small animal practice. Reviewing the illustrated cases with the text provides another avenue for learning and understanding this diagnostic specialty, because nothing can substitute for experience in film reading gained by case studies. It is suggested that the Atlas is used as an adviser and, as such, should be given a place near the radiographic viewbox, within easy reach when guidance is needed in film interpretation.

Emphasis is placed on illustrations of cases that provide examples of certain radiographic principles and patterns, and the Atlas should be used with this in mind, since it is not possible to include examples of all radiographic abnormalities seen in traumatized animals. This would be a completely different method of radiographic diagnostic interpretation, the "Aunt Minnie" approach. This method suggests that if one examines sufficient radiographs and memorizes the appearances of all of these, one will be adequately prepared for the next traumatized animal that comes to the clinic. However, this system does not function satisfactorily because it can be taken for granted that the radiographs of the next patient will be different from any one has ever seen before.

Consequently, one must rely on the detection and understanding of radiographic patterns that are made up of radiographic changes ("roentgen signs") as a result of various pathophysiological abnormalities. Therefore, it is strongly advised to work on the recognition of these patterns and then, most importantly, to discover how they developed and what they represent. Only then can one become comfortable with radiographs that conceal yet may reveal so much vital information if one will only take note.

In many cases, two orthogonal radiographic views are provided. When a second view does not really alter the radiographic interpretation, it is omitted. When a second view was unobtainable, an explanation is given. All lateral radiographs of the thorax and abdomen are reproduced with the head of the animal pointing to the left. All dorsoventral (thorax) and ventrodorsal (abdomen) radiographs are reproduced in ventrodorsal projection, with the animal's head at the top of the page. This means that the right side of the animal is at the left side of the page. The cases illustrated were originally examined at the Veterinary Medical Teaching Hospital, School of Veterinary Medicine, University of California, Davis, and the Department of Radiology, Faculty of Veterinary Medicine, University of Utrecht. This Atlas represents a joining together of the experiences drawn from the careers of two long-time colleagues who have enjoyed the times they spent together both professionally and socially. The authors acknowledge with gratitude all the many professional colleagues, faculty members and residents, who have directly and indirectly contributed to the information presented in the Atlas. Finally, a special word of recognition is reserved for the technical abilities and expertise of the many radiographers and photographers without whom this Atlas would not have been possible. Remember, without a diagnostic radiograph it is not possible to make an accurate diagnosis. Our thanks go out to that group of often unrecognized professionals.

The Authors

I. GENERAL INTRODUCTION

Trauma can be defined as physical force suddenly applied that results in anatomic and physiologic alterations. The severity of the changes varies with the amount of force applied, the means by which it is applied, and the anatomic location of its application. A traumatic event can mildly affect only a small portion of the animal's body and cause only mild discomfort, or it can severely affect multiple body areas and disrupt the function of vital organ systems. Before one can understand the effects of trauma on any part of the body, it must be realized that it is the number and severity of the associated injuries that usually determine the ultimate outcome. The true lethality of any particular injury can only be evaluated accurately when these factors are considered.

Trauma is an important health hazard to animals. A considerable percentage of animals presented to small animal clinicians arrive following a traumatic event. Many have sustained severe injury, and mortality rates are high due to spontaneous death or due to euthanasia requested or recommended because of the severity of the injury. For this reason, it is important to understand the use of radiology as a diagnostic and prognostic aid and to learn how to use it to the greatest advantage.

The most frequent causes of trauma include traffic accidents in which the animals are struck by a bicycle, motorbike, car, or truck, or have a wheel pass over the body, or are dragged some distance by the vehicle. Animals involved in fights with other animals constitute another large group of animals with the injury usually due to bite wounds. In the event of big dog-small dog interactions, the smaller animal may be "shaken" severely in addition to receiving multiple puncture wounds. Animals falling from heights may include those living in large cities with the injury resulting from a fall out of an apartment window high above the adjacent road or walkway. Other injuries of a similar type result from animals jumping into deep ditches or falling while walking in hilly regions. Crushing injuries occur to smaller animals when household items inadvert-

ently fall on them causing serious injury. Penetrating injuries occur commonly and are somewhat dependent on the nature of the surrounding society. The lesion can result from a variety of gunshot wounds or puncture wounds from sharp objects or from impalement. Unfortunately, human abuse is an increasingly frequent cause of trauma to animals and includes almost unimaginable types of injury. Without a history suggestive of trauma, the clinician is reminded to place trauma on the list of possible etiologies until more is understood about the animal's problems.

It is imperative that the veterinarian at the time of presentation be in a position to administer prompt treatment to avoid a fatal outcome in the ensuing hours or days after the injury. Owing to the vital nature of many of the body organs, these disruptive injuries can be rapidly fatal often before administration of treatment. This is obvious when considering that many of these animals die prior to arrival at the clinic. The animals that survive long enough to receive emergency treatment by the veterinarian have probably survived the most critical period of time relative to the injury and have a good chance for continued survival if accurately diagnosed and treated.

Radiology is an important diagnostic tool in the evaluation of the traumatized animal. The amount of time and money invested in this procedure can be substantial and priorities assigned to the radiographic examinations are often applied arbitrarily. It is not uncommon that a traumatized animal is radiographed for fractures and luxations, while no consideration is given to evaluation of the thoracic or abdominal regions. Rarely does the traumatized animal die of a fractured femur. However death due to peritoneal bleeding or due to an unsuspected diaphragmatic hernia is not so uncommon. This failure to radiograph the thorax and abdomen of the traumatized animal is astonishing because it has been clearly demonstrated so often that in animals with serious injury such as pneumothorax, diaphragmatic rupture, intra-abdominal hemorrhage, or urinary bladder rupture only minimal clinical signs may be present and the particular lesion not considered until radiographic evaluation. That is to say, it is imperative to search for the life-threatening injury present within the traumatized animal.

> **It is therefore important to emphasize from the very outset the main benefits of the radiographic examination of traumatized animals. Radiography assists the clinician in the following areas:**
>
> 1. recognition of cause and extent of life-threatening conditions in more detail than is possible by physical examination only (Fig. 1-1),
> 2. discrimination of the most serious condition for immediate treatment when multiple injuries are present (Fig. 1-2),
> 3. reassessment of the effectiveness of emergency therapy if the improvement of the animal is less than would be expected (Fig. 1-3),
> 4. provision of a permanent record that may be used as a basis for continued evaluation of the progress of the animal's recovery (Fig. 1-4).
>
> In this respect, it is important to emphasize that the exclusion of abnormalities is as important as the positive proof of their existence!

The timing of the radiographic examination in the course of early treatment of the traumatized animal is important. Radiography usually necessitates a compromise between the need for the information that might be gained from the radiographic examination and the stress applied to the animal in obtaining this. Life-threatening respiratory and circulatory emergencies or intra-abdominal injuries must be controlled and the animal's vital signs must be stabilized before a radiographic examination should be considered. Positioning and manipulation of the animal may be definitely contraindicated in the early stages of treatment.

> **The radiographic studies should be delayed if:**
>
> 1. the animal's condition could be aggravated by the radiographic procedures,
> 2. the expected benefits of radiography do not exceed the risk,
> 3. probable change in the course of therapy is unlikely.

A single lateral study can be made of most traumatized animals without great risk to the animal and important information can be derived from this study even though it is not a complete one. Remember that it is important to eventually complete the radiographic study by making the complementary orthogonal view as soon as is feasible. This is particularly important in thoracic trauma emergencies, in which a single lateral view alone can be misleading and conceal important information. If the orthogonal view can-

not be made in a routine manner because of restrictions in animal positioning, it is possible to consider use of a horizontal X-ray beam projection (Fig. 1-5). This is additionally helpful especially when looking for the presence of free air or fluid due to pneumothorax, pleural effusion, or pneumoperitoneum. Animals with suspected vertebral trauma should be radiographed as early as possible to determine the care that must be provided to stabilize the vertebral fracture/luxation. In animals of this type, the orthogonal view should be made by using a horizontal beam in order to avoid ventrodorsal positioning with the animal on its back.

Manipulation of the traumatized animal with fractures of bones in the extremities may not be life-threatening. However, the nature of the fracture can be altered by worsening the level of comminution or by additional soft tissue injury.

It may be necessary to use appropriate sedation or anesthesia if the level of pain precludes obtaining satisfactory radiographs. In this situation, it is important to be prepared for emergency assistance during the examination, and intubation of the animal should either be performed prior to the examination or should be readily available.

1. Importance of Radiographic Quality

Poor radiographic quality due to technical error(s) greatly increases the possibility of incorrect film evaluation. This is a particular problem with the traumatized animal because there may be difficulties in positioning or in completing the radiographic study. There is a natural tendency to avoid repeating radiographic studies on a traumatized animal and to deny that non-diagnostic radiographs have been produced. It is not uncommon when evaluating poor-quality radiographs to over-interpret shadows due to dirt on the animal's hair coat and call an artifact a lesion, or to call a normal anatomical variation on an oblique study a lesion, resulting in a false-positive evaluation. More often, however, the technical error prevents visualization of a lesion, causing a false-negative evaluation.

The effect of animal positioning is of obvious importance. Radiographic evaluation of the thorax and abdomen in the traumatized animal requires use of both a lateral and a ventrodorsal (VD) or dorsoventral (DV) projection. However, the selection of which lateral projection will be used or whether a DV or VD projection will be made often depends on the character of the injury and how the animal can most comfortably be positioned.

Comparison of the VD and DV views of the thorax shows a remarkable difference in the appearance of the diaphragm (Fig. 1-6). On the DV view, the X-ray beam intersects the diaphragm at nearly a right angle to the surface of the diaphragm; thus, the distance between the shadow of the ventral portion of the diaphragm and the two dorsally located crura is usually equal to the length of 3 to 4 vertebral bodies. On the VD view, the X-ray beam intersects the diaphragm almost parallel to its plane; thus, the distance between the shadow cast by the ventral portion of the diaphragm and the dorsally located crura is short and usually less than the length of 1 vertebral body. The cardiac silhouette also varies between the DV and VD views. The heart "falls" laterally when a deep-chested animal is placed in dorsal recumbency creating an elongated cardiac silhouette. On the DV view, the heart "hangs" in a more normal position and has an oblique "tear-drop-shaped" silhouette. Choice of a VD or DV view of the abdomen is less important and is usually determined by what is most comfortable for the traumatized animal. The DV view shows a gas-filled fundus of the stomach. On the VD view, the gas has moved and outlines the pylorus and descending duodenum (Fig. 1-7).

Regardless of the view, almost all thoracic studies of small animals are made with the animal in recumbent position. That means that the lower lung is compressed and contains little air. As a result, little contrast remains between the lung lesion and the surrounding healthy lung to permit identification of either infiltrative or space-occupying pulmonary masses. The compression of the dependent lung is caused by pressure of the abdominal contents on the diaphragm, the weight of the heart, and the pressure of the tabletop against the lower rib cage, preventing its expansion. Thus, a comparison of right and left lateral views, or VD and DV views, always permits visualization of the lung in a manner that provides for more complete evaluation than when only a single view is used. The character of the suspected lesion may influence the choice by which view the lesion is best evaluated. The choice of a right or left lateral abdominal study is of less importance (Fig. 1-8).

Rotation of the animal in a lateral thoracic study results in superimposition of a part of the dorsal lung field by the vertebral column. Obliquity of the DV/VD view makes the cardiac silhouette appear larger and displaces the vertebral column laterally, resulting in partial obscuring of one lung field whereas the other lung field is seen to a greater extent. Obliquity resulting from poor positioning of the animal for an abdominal study is less important since the abdominal organs move freely within the abdominal cavity and do not have a fixed location or radiographic appearance.

2. Characteristics of a Diagnostic Study

Standard positioning for a complete radiographic study of the thorax or abdomen includes one lateral and either a VD or DV projection. For extremities, two orthogonal projections are used. Most clinicians are more familiar with the appearance of the right lateral radiograph of the thorax and select this lateral view. In the traumatized animal, it is usually less stressful to obtain straight positioning of the thorax by using sternal recumbency (DV) with the forelegs extended cranially. Unfortunately, this does not enable full expansion of the rib cage to obtain as good an inspiratory film as can be obtained in the VD position. For abdominal radiography, most clinicians are familiar with the appearance of the right lateral radiograph. In the traumatized animal, either lateral view is acceptable with the knowledge that the left lateral view is more helpful in the evaluation of the pylorus and duodenum (Fig. 1-8).

Instead of obtaining a second orthogonal view, only one single recumbent lateral view is erroneously used for evaluation of trauma animals. This is a most serious technical error. This text includes examples of lateral projections which have been proven to be inadequate for complete diagnosis. As an example, it may be necessary to take both right and left recumbent lateral views of the thorax in defining a lesion that is first only identified on the DV or VD view.

Improper cassette size often compromises a thoracic study when cassettes are used that are not large enough to permit evaluation of the complete thorax, including the thoracic inlet and the entire diaphragm. To obtain the best lateral thoracic study, the primary beam must be centered on the heart and the shoulders and front legs must be positioned cranially so that they are not superimposed over the cranial aspects of the lung fields. By positioning the head and neck in slight extension, the cranial aspect of the thoracic cavity, including the trachea, is seen more clearly. Both the diaphragm and pelvic region should be included in studies of the abdomen and failure to include them brings on an incomplete study since these two anatomical regions are so frequently affected in traumatized animals. In extremital studies, an attempt should be made to include both ends of a traumatized bone to ensure complete evaluation of the injury. Use of a lateral projection of the entire limb made on a large film is a good technique for a survey study, but it should be completed prior to surgery on the anesthetized animal.

Use of correct exposure factors is an absolute necessity for a good study of the traumatized animal. Incorrect settings may be a frequent technical problem because of inaccurate measuring of the animal. A technique chart should recommend use of: (1) the highest possible kVp to allow for use of a decreased mAs, (2) the highest mA, and (3) the shortest possible exposure time settings. This ensures that an X-ray machine with sufficient capacity is being used correctly, and is producing the highest quality radiographs possible. High kVp settings reduce radiographic contrast, ensuring a relatively gray film with low contrast differences between the different tissue densities. This technique is used for thoracic radiography. Lower kVp settings result in radiographs with higher contrast. This technique is more suitable for abdominal radiography. Errors in technique selection may be related to machine limits, in which instance it must be realized that the X-ray machine or imaging system (cassette, screens and film) does not have adequate capability, particularly for thoracic radiography. With dyspnea following trauma, thoracic contents move rapidly and an exposure time of 1/30 of a second or less is necessary to reliably prevent blurring (motion artifact) on a thoracic study. A longer exposure time results in movement of the lungs and degradation of radiographic detail in the radiograph. Use of a combination of faster rare-earth-type intensifying screens and appropriate film reduces the required radiographic exposure and is an alternative to obtaining a more powerful machine. Radiography of the abdomen or musculoskeletal structures is easier because these structures don't move so much. For those studies, a slower film-screen combination or the faster system that is used for thoracic radiography may be chosen. For these studies, a lower kVp setting of around 70 kVp is used.

The appropriate use of a grid contributes greatly to improvement of the image quality of the film. It should be used with animals having a thoracic measurement greater than 15 cm or an abdominal measurement greater than 11 cm. It is extremely important to use a grid in traumatized animals because of the likelihood of pleural, pulmonary or peritoneal hemorrhage that increases tissue density and results in scatter radiation. The grid removes much of the scatter radiation that produces fogging of the film with resulting loss of contrast.

Grids may be used in either a stationary mode, whereby the grid lines are seen on the radiograph, or in an oscillating mode that moves the grid during the exposure time and blurs the grid lines so that they are not identified on the resulting radiograph. A fine-line stationary grid has visible grid lines which do not significantly reduce image sharpness. This type of grid is more suitable to use with the short exposure times required in thoracic radiography of the traumatized animal, since the older type of oscillating grids do not move quickly enough to blur the grid lines, resulting in prominent grid lines still visible on the radiograph.

The best film-screen combination for thoracic radiography of the traumatized animal, in the event that the X-ray machine has only limited power, is one of the fast rare-earth-type screens with a matching high-latitude film. This permits use of shorter exposure times up to 1/6 of that previously used and produces low-contrast radiographs without motion artifacts.

These high-speed systems produce radiographs that may appear somewhat grainy, with some loss of detail or sharp-

ness compared with a finer-grain screen; however, the loss of detail due to the use of the high-speed systems is less than the loss in detail due to the effects caused by motion unsharpness. While an important problem in thoracic radiography, choice of film-screen combinations for abdominal and extremity radiography is not as critical because of the decreased chance of animal movement during the exposure.

If the X-ray machine is of a higher rating, one has the choice of selecting a slower-speed screen while still achieving an adequate radiographic exposure with a short exposure time. Use of the slower-speed system improves radiographic quality since the resulting radiograph is much less grainy.

The intensifying screens must be free of surface artifacts caused by dirt or spillage of processing solutions. Many of these screen artifacts can be removed by simply cleaning the surface of the screens. However, if they remain over a period of time, they become permanent, causing an artifact that is repeated on every radiograph made with that cassette.

3. Radiographic Evaluation

There are two basic methods of film evaluation. The first technique is to "memorize" the appearance of the disease or pathologic changes that you expect to be present, and then examine the radiograph looking carefully for those features. This is the approach taken by traditional textbooks of medicine, which present diseases with a description and an illustration of the typical radiological appearance. The difficulty with this approach is similar to the difficulty found in applying textbook knowledge to the reality of a sick animal. Clinical information of the traumatized animal is often indefinite and ambiguous. It is the same with the information available from a radiograph. In many animals, the radiologic picture of a disease is not "typical", and the textbook approach therefore leads to confusion or misdiagnosis.

The second method of film evaluation uses the "radiographic sign" method. This is a much more accurate method of film evaluation. It involves examination of the films, searching for pathophysiological changes shown by these particular radiological "signs", and then relating them to various conditions that are known to cause them. As there are often many signs on a radiograph involving more than one organ, a systematic analysis using deductive reasoning leads to an appropriate differential diagnosis.

Successful evaluation of the radiograph must be systematic in order to ensure that all parts of the radiograph are completely examined. This means that one needs to devise a system for film evaluation that follows either the anatomical character of the study, or the physical character of the radiograph.

Use of the anatomical technique requires that each organ that can be seen on the radiograph is looked for and evaluated.

The physical examination technique begins with examination of the peripheral strucures and is followed by successive steps of decreasing the field of vision until the central region of the film is reached.

The greatest error in film evaluation of a traumatized animal is to immediately look for the lesion expected following one's physical examination. This leads to missing all of the other important information contained on the radiograph.

In this book, for the purpose of examination the animal's body is divided into three regions: the thorax, the abdomen, and the musculoskeletal system. While this provides a convenient method of presentation, it is important to remember that it is not uncommon for a traumatic incident to have caused injury to more than one region in the body. Multiple radiographic studies are often required.

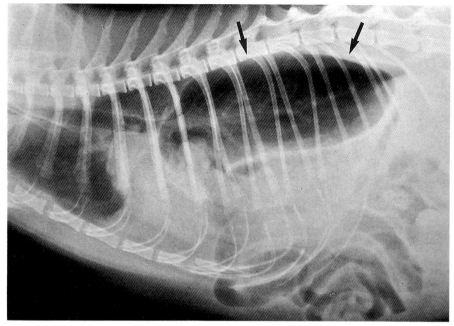

A

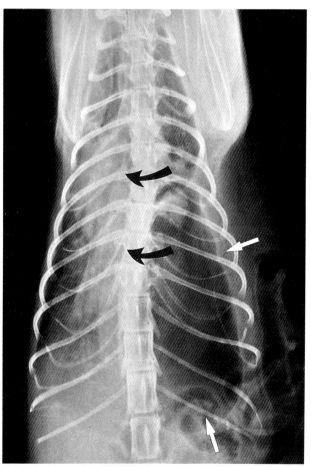

B

Figure 1-1.
Paracostal hernia, in combination with diaphragmatic hernia.
By physical examination of this traumatized 5-year-old domestic short-haired cat, a paracostal hernia with displacement of small bowel loops into the subcutaneous rupture was evident. However, the severity of possible intrathoracic abnormalities could only be assumed. Thoracic radiographs revealed an additional diaphragmatic hernia, with presence of a gas-filled stomach (straight arrows) in the left hemithorax and displacement of the mediastinum and heart (curved arrows) to the right side as seen on the dorsoventral view.

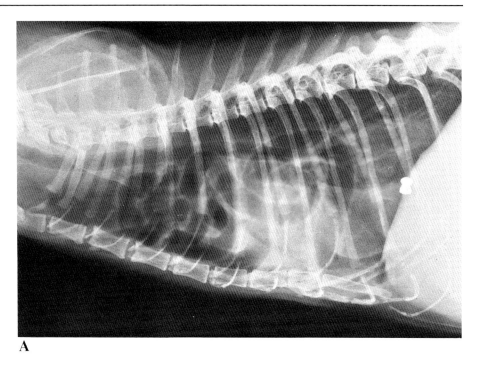

A

Figure 1-2.

Diaphragmatic hernia, in combination with gastric dilatation and volvulus.

*A 3-year-old domestic short-haired cat was presented with clinical signs of dyspnea and severe abdominal distension after being hit by a car. Thoracic radiographs revealed the presence of small bowel loops in the left hemithorax indicating diaphragmatic hernia (**A**). Additional abdominal films revealed a severely distended and gas-filled stomach in a volvulus position (**B**). Due to the displacement of the small bowel loops through the left-sided diaphragmatic rupture, the gastric antrum (arrow) and duodenum had been pulled over to the left side and had become occluded. Swallowing of air had resulted in life-threatening gastric distension.*

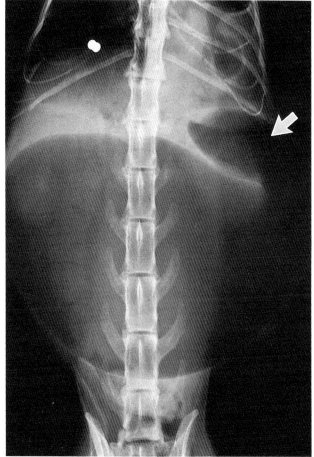

B

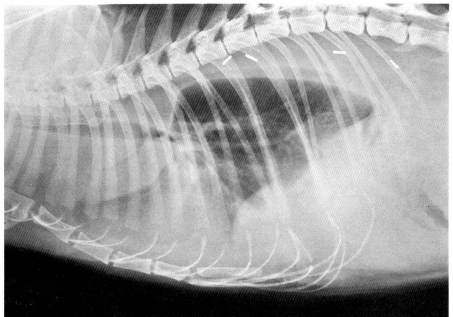

Figure 1-3.
Chylothorax, recurrence after reparative surgery.
Following a traffic accident, this 10-year-old domestic short-haired cat had developed severe dyspnea. A chylothorax due to thoracic duct rupture was diagnosed and thoracic surgery with closing of the duct had been performed successfully. However, after 3 days the cat became dyspneic again. Thoracic radiographs revealed severe pleural effusion with compression-atelectasis of the cranial and middle lung lobes.

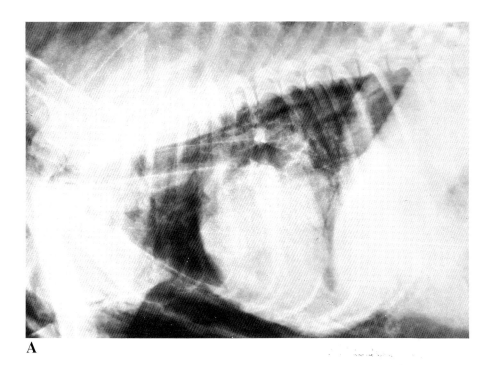

A

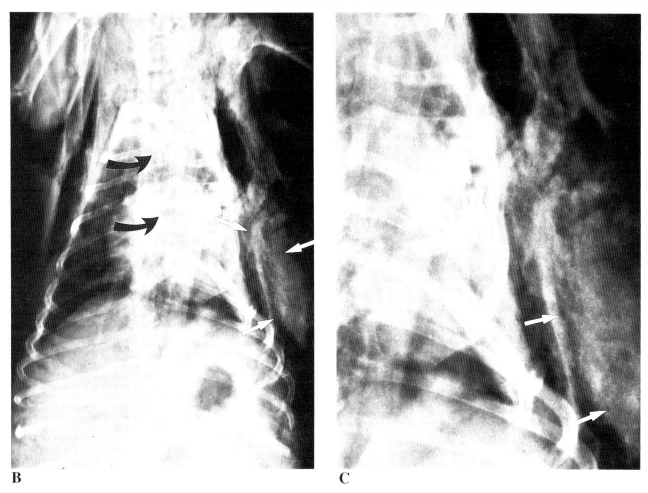

B

C

Figure 1-4.
Flail chest, with exteriorization of a lung lobe.
A 3-year-old Samoyed was hit by a motorbike and presented very dyspneic, in shock, with laboured breathing, and a flail segment in the left thoracic wall. Clinical investigation revealed considerable subcutaneous emphysema and the presence of rib fractures, in combination with a soft tissue mass in the left thoracic wall. Due to the animal's distress, only one lateral radiograph was made (A). This film did not present much additional information concerning the severity or character of the thoracic lesions. Following administration of fluid therapy, additional dorsoventral radiographs were made (B, C). These films presented more accurate information of the status of the thorax. Four adjacent ribs of the left thoracic wall (ribs 4-7) were crushed and dislocated. The heart was obviously displaced to the left and was in contact with the fractured ribs. Also, the trachea was displaced to the left (curved arrows). Outside the rib-cage, a well-circumscribed soft tissue mass was visible that is outlined by subcutaneous gas (straight arrows). At surgery, this proved to be the left cranial lung lobe that had herni- ated through the chest wall interruption.

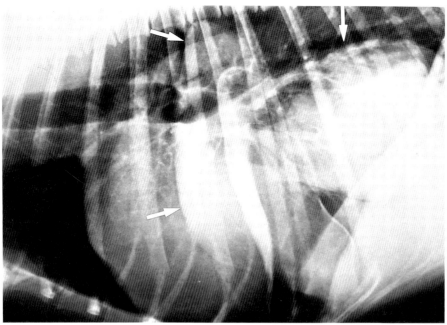

A

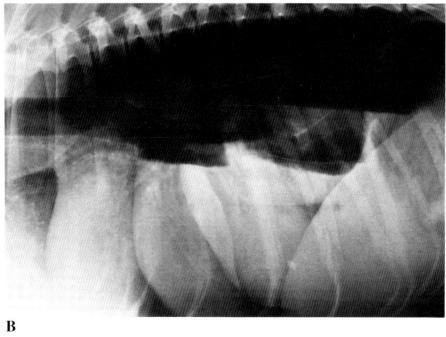

B

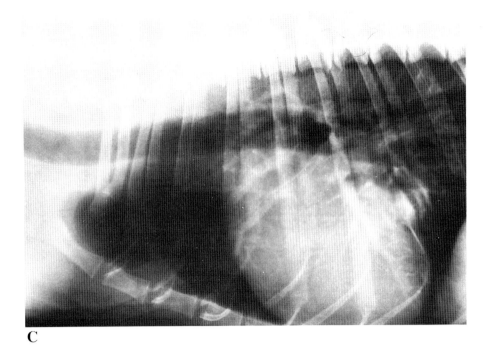

C

Figure 1-5.
Pulmonary pseudocysts (pneumatoceles).
*Twelve days after being hit by a car, this 5-year-old Hovawarth was presented for ra-diographic examination of the thorax. The lateral recumbent film (**A**) showed several localized, well-circumscribed fluid-dense structures (arrows) that seemed to be con-tained within the lung lobes. A horizontal beam projection with the dog in a standing position (**B**) revealed gas-fluid levels in these structures. These changes are radio-graphic signs of traumatic pulmonary pseudocysts, filled with a combination of blood and air. After 6 weeks, the pseudocysts had resolved completely and the radiographic presentation of the thorax had returned to normal (**C**).*

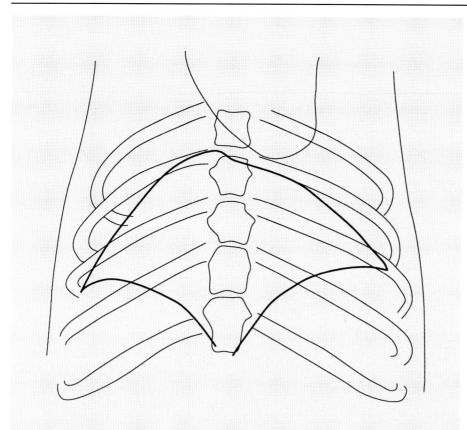

Figure 1-6.
Drawings of the diaphragm.
These drawings illustrate the re-markable difference in the ra-diographic appearance of the diaphragm when viewed dor-soventrally **(A),** *when the X-ray beam intersects the diaphragm at a right angle, and ventro-dorsally* **(B),** *when the X-ray beam intersects the diphragm in a parallel manner.*

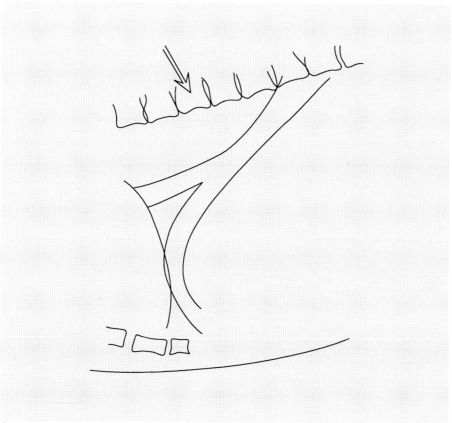

A

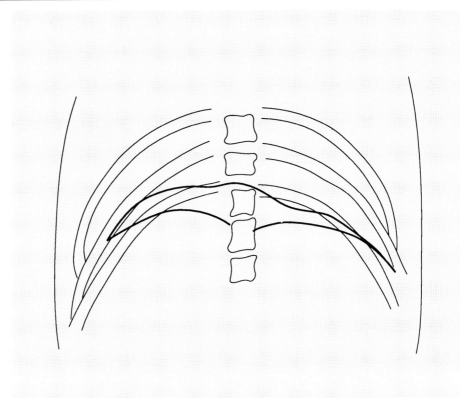

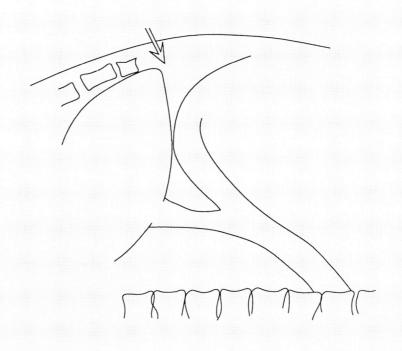

B

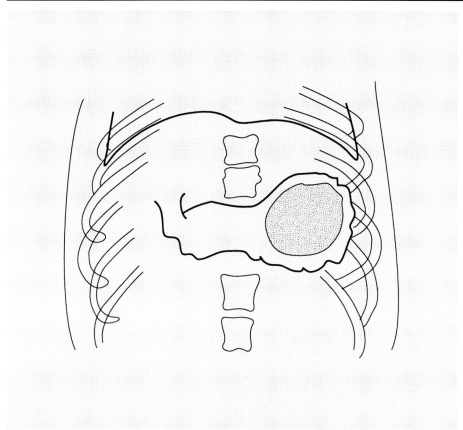

A

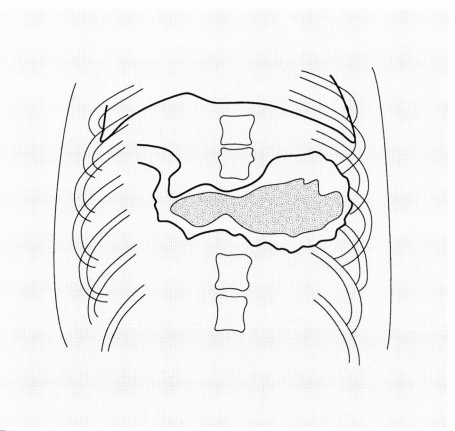

B

Figure 1-7.
Drawings of the stomach.
*These drawings illustrate differences in appearance of the stomach. In the dorsoventral view (**A**), the air fills the fundus while in the ventrodorsal view (**B**), the air fills the pyloric antrum and duodenum.*

Figure 1-8.
Drawings of the stomach.
*These drawings illustrate differences in appearance of the stomach. In the right lateral view (**A**), the air fills the fundus while in the left lateral view (**B**), the air fills the pyloric antrum and duodenum.*

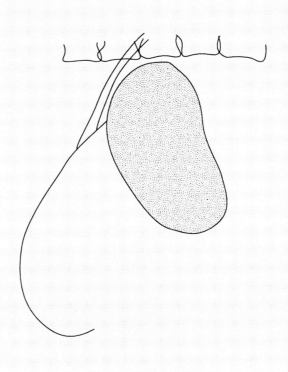

A

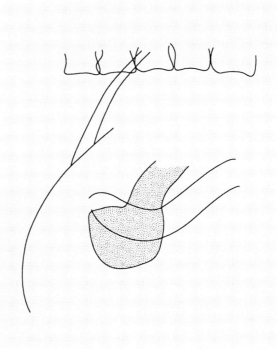

B

II. RADIOLOGY OF THORACIC TRAUMA

1. Introduction

Radiology is a most important diagnostic tool in the investigation of thoracic trauma because it reveals more specific information than physical examination and can be performed relatively cheaply, quickly, and safely, providing rapid results on which to base decisions relative to diagnosis and/or treatment. The X-ray image is a transillumination of the body at the moment the film is made. It is this ability to see a representation of the interior of the animal, impossible by palpation or auscultation, that accounts for the great value of thoracic radiography. The good contrast provided by the air in the lungs opens up a window to the thoracic organs on survey radiographs to an extent not possible with abdominal radiographic studies.

Accurate radiographic diagnosis is vital because physical signs of thoracic organ dysfunction following trauma are often ambiguous. In addition, radiographic examination provides a temporal dimension to evaluate a progression of changes as they are found in the course of the disease. Radiographs reproduce the character of the animal's thorax on film which can be examined both at the time of the original examination as well as later.

Because the lung is largely composed of air, it normally appears relatively dark (radiolucent) on a normally exposed film. Increased lung density is due to either decrease in air content or increase in fluid content. As a result, the lungs are whiter than normal (increased lung opacity). This is a common finding in the traumatized dog or cat due to pulmonary hemorrhage. It is also possible for the lung to become more radiolucent following trauma. Now the lungs are blacker than normal (decreased lung density/opacity). This occurs in a hypovolemic situation. A problem in determining lung opacity occurs in animals with diffuse or generalized patterns that present little opportunity to make a comparison between diseased and normal lung opacity.

While thoracic injuries are common and often life-threatening, the thorax and its contents are not as easily injured as might be expected. The thorax is tough and resilient due to its strong, spring-like ribs. The lungs add protection against impact to the heart through their air-cushion effect. Because of these protections, virtually all thoracic injuries are due to high-energy forces generated by violent trauma. Consequently, thoracic injuries are often part of a constellation of injuries involving several areas of the animal's body. While the radiographic study often provides specific information at the time of the trauma, it is also important in following the healing process, providing information about changes that appear secondarily at a later point of time. A late developing mediastinal hemorrhage is an example of this type of injury. The radiographic study may also serve as a preanesthesia study for older animals or when cardiac disease is suspected. More specific reasons for thoracic radiography include evaluation of known or suspected non-cardiogenic edema following several types of uncommon trauma such as:
– electrical shock,
– near-drowning,
– head trauma, or
– near-asphyxiation.

2. Radiographic Appearance of the Normal Thorax

The most fundamental diagnostic decision is to determine if the radiographs are of a normal or abnormal thorax, and this is often the most difficult decision to make (Fig. 2-1). The canine thorax is highly variable because of age and breed differences. Breed and the age of the patient affect body conformation and are important causes of variability. Puppies, mature and old animals with aging changes have markedly different radiographic appearances. Degenerative changes without clinical significance such as lung fibrosis or calcified costal cartilage may closely resemble clinically important lesions seen in the traumatized dog (Fig. 2-1).

The stage of respiration greatly influences the radiographic appearance of the thorax and may be difficult to control in the trauma patient. A film exposed in expiration has significantly different features when compared with those exposed at full inspiration. If not appreciated, these differences are great enough to cause misdiagnosis of lung disease. At expiration, the lungs are relatively more radiopaque and smaller in size, with a decreased angle between the diaphragm and spine on the lateral view and between the diaphragm and thoracic wall on the DV or VD view. The triangle formed by the caudal border of the heart, the ventral portion of the diaphragm, and the caudal vena cava is smaller on expiration. Also, the diaphragm is more cranial and convex and has greater contact with the heart which appears relatively larger on the expiratory film because of the diminished size of the thoracic cavity; meanwhile, the ribs are closer together and at a greater angle with the spine (Fig. 2-2).

Obesity is common, particularly in older animals, and creates an overall increased opacity because of the greater amount of soft tissue. Increased lung opacity is also caused by poor lung inflation since obese animals rarely breathe deeply. As a result, it is most of the time impossible to make good thoracic films due to inadequate lung inflation. The resulting underexposure can lead to a false diagnosis of lung disease because the artifactual increased lung density strongly resembles a diffuse pulmonary infiltrate that might be associated with pulmonary hemorrhage.

3. Radiographic Changes due to Thoracic Trauma

Having decided that the thoracic radiographs indicate abnormalities, the next question is to determine the character of the injury and the clinical significance of the pathological change. This can be most easily done by evaluating the thorax in a categorical manner.

Structural damage to the thorax caused by trauma can most easily be divided into five categories:

1. disruption of the thoracic wall (bellows apparatus)
2. fluid or air in the pleural space
3. diaphragmatic rupture ("diaphragmatic hernia")
5. damage to the lung parenchyma
6. mediastinal injury (heart, great vessels, thoracic duct, and esophagus).

3.1. Disruption of the thoracic wall (bellows apparatus)

The traumatized chest wall often has lesions due to injury to the soft tissues and ribs (Table 2-1). Radiography will help to define and evaluate the extent of underlying damage. Injury of the chest wall results in diminished efficiency of respiration and restricted expansion of the rib cage. Skeletal structures may be injured and examination of the vertebrae, costo-vertebral articulations, sternebrae, ribs, costal arches, costochondral junctions, scapulae, and the proximal part of the forelimbs must be focused on the detection of fractures or dislocations. Furthermore, radiographs prove very helpful for evaluation of secondary changes, such as open chest wounds, secondary lung compression, pulmonary and/or mediastinal hemorrhage, pleural fluid, adhesions, diaphragmatic rupture with displacement and/or incarceration of the viscera asociated with diaphragmatic rupture.

Flail chest is a unique injury in which there are proximal and distal fractures of consecutive ribs, resulting in a section of the thoracic wall that is free to move independently and paradoxically during breathing. Presence of this loose section of thoracic wall ("flail segment") is usually accompanied by pneumothorax and by damage to the adjacent lung (pulmonary contusion) and results in severe ventilatory compromise (Figs. 1-4, 2-3).

Table 2-1:
Radiographic signs of thoracic wall injury

1. soft tissue swelling (Fig. 2-3)
2. subcutaneous emphysema (Figs. 1-4, 2-3)
3. malaligned rib fragments (fractured ribs (Figs. 1-4, 2-3)
4. malpositioned ribs (intercostal muscle tear) (Fig. 2-3)
5. underlying pleural fluid (hemorrhage)
6. lung retraction (pleural air) (Fig. 2-3)
7. lung contusion (hemorrhage) (Fig. 2-3)
8. vertebral or sternal fractures

3.2. Fluid or air in the pleural space

Injury resulting in fluid or air in the pleural space can be caused by penetrating trauma to the thoracic wall or by blunt trauma to the thorax while the glottis is closed. In the normal dog or cat, the pleural space is usually not visible on radiographs; however, in the traumatized animal, this normally minimal space may be filled with fluid (pleural effusion) or air (pneumothorax) or may contain abdominal viscera (diaphragmatic hernia). Examination of any pleural lesion is important to determine if it has a generalized or focal location. Determination of whether the pleural fluid or air is stationary or movable assists in understanding more of the duration of the lesion, its pathogenesis, and its charact. The character of the pleural lesion can be studied by radiographing the animal in varying positions.

Pneumothorax is the collection of free air within the pleural space, resulting in a loss of intrathoracic negative pressure, thus allowing the lungs to recoil away from the thoracic wall. Radiographic changes of pneumothorax are one of the most common sequelae to thoracic trauma and can be found with penetrating chest wall injuries or, more commonly, with rupture of the lung parenchyma or bronchi when the chest wall is intact (Table 2-2). Usually, the pneumothorax is bilateral because the thin mediastinum ruptures easily at the time of the original trauma; however, it may be unilateral.

Table 2-2: **Radiographic signs of pneumothorax**

1. increased size and lucency of the thoracic cavity (both views) (Figs. 2-4, 2-6, 2-8)
2. separation of cardiac apex from the sternum (lateral view) (Figs. 2-4, 2-8)
3. retraction of pulmonary borders from the thoracic wall (both views) (Figs. 2-4, 2-5, 2-6, 2-7, 2-8)
4. vascular and bronchial shadows do not extend to the chest wall (both views) (Figs. 2-4, 2-5, 2-7, 2-8)
5. increased density of lung lobes due to partial collapse (both views) (Figs. 2-4, 2-5, 2-6, 2-8)
6. caudal displacement of diaphragm (lateral view) (Figs. 2-4,2-9)
7. flattened diaphragm (lateral view) (Figs. 2-4, 2-8, 2-9)
8. mediastinal shift (DV/VD views) (Fig. 2-7)

Tension pneumothorax results from an injury that creates a valve-like lesion that permits filling of the pleural space with air on inspiration. Closure of the valve occurs on expiration resulting in progressive filling of the pleural space with air. The lungs collapse, the mediastinum shifts away from the side with the tension pneumothorax, the diaphragm shifts caudally, and the chest cavity increases in size. This is a life-threatening condition (Fig. 2-11). Pseudo-pneumothorax can be seen radiographically due to superimposition of skin folds (Fig. 2-10).

Radiographic changes of pleural effusion show loss of the cardiac silhouette, loss of the diaphragmatic silhouette, retraction of the lung lobes, and visualization of the lung fissures (Table 2-3). The fluid is movable and can be changed in position remarkably between the DV and VD views. While the fluid is usually effusive, it may also be due to hemorrhage or rupture of the thoracic duct. Thoracocentesis is required to determine the character of the fluid.

Table 2-3:
Radiographs signs of pleural fluid (pleural effusion, hemothorax, chylothorax)

1. increased density of the thoracic cavity (both views) (Figs. 1-3, 2-12, 2-13)
2. retraction of the lung lobes from the thoracic wall (both views) (Fig. 1-3)
3. fluid-dense shadows between the thoracic wall and the lung lobes (both views) (Figs. 1-3, 2-13)
4. interlobar fissures and triangular fluid pockets at the peripheral portions of the interlobar fissures (DV or VD view) (Figs. 1-1, 1-3, 2-13)
5. blunting of the costodiaphragmatic angles with rounding of the peripheral lung lobe tips (DV or VD view) (Fig. 1-3)
6. positional changes of the fluid collections (both views)
7. indistinct heart shadow because of fluid pocket (both views) (Figs. 2-12, 2-13)
8. caudal displacement of flattened diaphragm (lateral view) (Figs. 1-3, 2-12)
9. heart shadow not visualized (both views) (Figs. 1-3, 2-12, 2-13)

3.3. Diaphragmatic rupture

Diaphragmatic rupture follows a forceful impact on the abdomen when the glottis is open and the lungs can collapse. Radiography is performed to diagnose and determine the presence of diaphragmatic injury and to localize the rupture site prior to surgical correction. In addition, the radiographs may identify pulmonary and/or mediastinal hemorrhage, pleural fluid, or fractures. Radiographic changes associated with a diaphragmatic hernia include loss of the diaphragmatic silhouette, absence of the normal caudal silhouette of the heart, and increased density in the caudal thoracic regions. The liver may not be identifiable within the abdominal cavity, and the stomach and duodenum may be displaced from their normal position. Gas-filled intestinal loops may be detected inside the thoracic cavity. Pleural effusion occurs due to constriction by the contracting diaphragmatic tear with resulting entrapment of a liver lobe or small bowel loop(s). If the stomach becomes lodged within the thoracic cavity and the pylorus becomes occluded, gastric dilatation may occur (Table 2-4).

In cases of doubt, an oral barium follow-through study can be performed to demonstrate the presence of concealed gastrointestinal segments inside the thoracic cavity or to demonstrate minor dislocations of the gastric antrum and duodenum within the cranial abdomen.

Lesions that make identification of the diaphragm very difficult include pulmonary masses that silhouette with the diaphragm, pleural fluid adjacent to the diaphragm, or cau-

Table 2-4:
Radiographic signs of traumatic diaphragmatic hernia

1. incomplete diaphragmatic silhouette (both views) (Figs. 1-2, 2-9, 2-14, 2-15, 2-16, 2-17, 2-18, 2-19, 2-20)
2. partially or completely obscured cardiac silhouette (both views) (Figs. 1-2, 2-15, 2-16, 2-17, 2-18, 2-20, 2-21)
3. asymmetry of diaphragmatic outline (DV view) (Fig. 2-15)
4. altered slope of diaphragm (lateral view) (Figs. 2-15, 2-17, 2-20)
5. pleural effusion (both views) (Figs. 2-15, 2-16, 2-18, 2-19)
6. abnormal intrathoracic structures, liver, spleen, omentum, with soft tissue density (both views) (Figs. 2-9, 2-15, 2-21)
7. abnormal intrathoracic structures with loculated gas pockets (both views) (Figs. 1-2, 2-17, 2-19, 2-20)
8. abnormal intrathoracic structures with granular-dense (fecal-like) material (both views) (Fig. 2-19)
9. displacement of lung lobes (both views) (Fig. 2-14)
10. displacement of heart and trachea (both views) (Figs. 1-1, 2-9, 2-14, 2-20)
11. fractures of ribs, sternal segments, vertebra, or scapula (both views) (Fig. 2-21)
12. subcutaneous emphysema (both views)
13. displacement of pyloric antrum and duodenal bulb (both abdominal views) (Figs. 2-18, 2-20)
14. gastric dilatation associated with gastric herniation (both views) (Figs. 1-1, 2-20)
15. disappearance of falciform fat triangle under liver in cats (lateral view) (Figs. 2-16, 2-20)
16. absence of abdominal viscera (both abdominal views) (Figs. 2-20, 2-22)

Table 2-5:
Differential diagnosis for diaphragmatic hernia

1. congenital peritoneo-pericardial hernia (Fig. 2-23)
2. congenital or acquired peritoneo-mediastinal hernia
3. sliding hiatal hernia
4. paraesophageal hiatal hernia (Fig. 2-24)
5. gastroesophageal intussusception
6. paracostal hernia (on lateral view) (Fig. 1-1)
7. pulmonary paraesophageal mass
8. pulmonary mass adjacent to diaphragm
9. pleural effusion adjacent to diaphragm
10. diaphragmatic paralysis with cranial displacement
11. subdiaphragmatic mass producing an abnormal diaphragmatic contour

3.4. Damage to the lung parenchyma

Damage to the lung parenchyma may be an independent lesion or may be associated with other injuries. Identification of bronchi, arteries and veins, and interlobar fissures directs the evaluation of each individual lobe. One technique of examination is to start the examination of the lungs centrally, to proceed to the mid-lung, and finally to examine the periphery of the lung, looking for any radiographic pattern that is different and thus, perhaps, indicative of disease. It is helpful to compare the appearance of right and left lung fields or adjacent lung lobes, looking especially for opacity, degree of inflation, and appearance of vascular structures within the lung. Configuration of the thorax may be deep and narrow, intermediate, or wide and shallow, and it may greatly influence the appearance of the lung fields. Lung fields of the traumatized animal frequently show pulmonary hemorrhage or bullae formation. Note that it is easier to visualize the pulmonary vessels and bronchi on the lateral view than on the DV view because the lungs in the DV view are often slightly overexposed.

Abnormalities to the lung parenchyma include increased pulmonary fluid (Table 2-6), lung rupture or laceration with formation of pulmonary hematomas (Table 2-7) or bullae formation (pneumatocele) (Table 2-8). Most animals with blunt thoracic trauma suffer some degree of pulmonary contusion, with edema and hemorrhage in the lung parenchyma. These types of injuries are caused by penetrating trauma to the thoracic wall or by blunt trauma to the thorax while the glottis is closed and an increased intrapulmonary pressure results. Pulmonary contusion is caused by rapid compression and subsequent decompression of the lungs, resulting in disruption of the alveolar-capillary integrity, thus causing a diffuse bruise of the underlying lung with consequent hemorrhage and edema of the alveolar and interstitial spaces. Pulmonary hematomas may be formed if localized bleeding is trapped within the

dal mediastinal masses. A particular differential diagnosis in patients suspected of having a traumatic diaphragmatic hernia is that of a congenital peritoneo-pericardial hernia in which abdominal viscera are located within the pericardial sac (Fig. 2-23). While many of the radiographic findings are similar to those seen in trauma cases, the absence of pleural fluid and the abnormally enlarged cardiac silhouette are suggestive signs of the congenital lesion. A sliding hiatal hernia or paraesophageal hiatal hernia (Fig. 2-24) or gastroesophageal intussusception create a mass lesion adjacent to the diaphragm just caudal to the heart shadow and resemble a small diaphragmatic hernia. Use of a barium swallow provides a clearer identification of these lesions. A differential diagnosis for diaphragmatic hernia is listed (Table 2-5).

pulmonary parenchyma, forming a fluid-dense pocket. Pulmonary cysts are presumed to represent a coalescence of ruptured airspaces within the lung parenchyma. They present as localized, spherical radiolucent lesions that are filled with air or with a combination of air and fluid.

Pulmonary rupture with leakage of air usually results in pneumothorax. Sometimes, it causes pneumomediastinum and associated pneumoretroperitoneum that can be recognized because of easier visualization on the radiograph of soft tissue structures that are contrasted by air within the mediastinum and retroperitoneal space. Pneumothorax is discussed as a pleural lesion.

Table 2-6:
Radiographic signs of increased pulmonary fluid (hemorrhage or edema)

1. lesions with lobular, lobar, or multiple lobe distribution (Figs. 2-25, 2-26, 2-27, 2-28, 2-29)
2. infiltrative pattern with indistinct borders (Figs. 2-25, 2-27)
3. location without special relationship to hilar region (Figs. 2-17, 2-28, 2-29, 2-30, 2-31)
4. lesions associated with chest wall injury (Figs. 2-3, 2-25)
5. air-bronchogram pattern indicating severe contusion (Figs. 2-26, 2-27)
6. increased lung density because of lung collapse secondary to pneumothorax (Figs. 2-3, 2-4, 2-5, 2-7, 2-8, 2-11)

Table 2-7:
Radiographic signs of pulmonary hematomas

1. usually more than one lesion in the same or adjacent lobes (Fig. 2-32)
2. nodular pattern with distinct borders (Fig. 2-32)
3. radiodensity due to hemorrhage
4. radiolucent center because of air plus hemorrhage
5. tendency for peripheral location in the lung lobe (Fig. 2-32)

Table 2-8:
Radiographic signs of pulmonary bullae

1. usually more than one lesion in the same or adjacent lobes (Figs. 1-5, 2-32, 2-33)
2. nodular pattern with thin border (Fig. 2-32)
3. radiolucent contents (Figs. 1-5, 2-32, 2-33)
4. usually peripheral in the lung lobe (Fig. 2-33)
5. thin discrete wall (Fig. 2-33)

It is possible for the lung density to be decreased rather than increased. This is a much less common finding, but is clinically important when noted. Thromboembolic lung disease results in a decrease in the amount of blood flowing to and through the lungs (Fig. 2-34). This disease causes occluding of multiple pulmonary vessels and often follows the original trauma with some time interval. It may be present in animals that do not recover as expected. In the more acutely injured patient, hypovolemia is a common finding. In addition to microcardia, the pulmonary vasculature is diminished in size and the lungs appear more radiolucent than usual (Fig. 2-35). Lung fields can also appear radiolucent following trauma due to the collapse of the lung lobes with an associated pneumothorax, especially a tension pneumothorax. Lung fields can also appear radiolucent because of overexposure making the chest appear empty (Fig. 2-35).

3.5. Mediastinal injury
Injury to the mediastinum may involve the heart, aorta, the air-filled trachea, esophagus, major vessels, and thymus or lymph nodes. The mediastinal space is divided into the cranial mediastinal space, which contains the trachea, esophagus, great vessels, thymus, and sternal and cranial mediastinal lymph nodes. The central mediastinal structures include principally the heart, esophagus, and the hilar region with its major vessels and lymph nodes. The caudal mediastinal structures include the esophagus and caudal vena cava.

Hemomediastinum is present when the mediastinum fills with blood as a result of trauma (Table 2-9). Hemomediastinum results in increased widening and density of the cranial mediastinal structures, both on lateral and dorsoventral films. This increased density is often overlooked on the first radiographic study at the time of early bleeding, but is more clearly identified on a second study made as the animal fails to recover as expected from the trauma. An associated hemopericardium causes an increase in the size of the cardiac silhouette on both views with marked rounding of the shadow.

Table 2-9:
Radiographic signs of hemomediastinum

1. increased density of the cranial mediastinal structures (lateral view) (Fig. 2-36)
2. widened mediastinal shadow (both views) (Fig. 2-36)
3. associated hemopericardium
4. decreased size of pulmonary vessels due to cardiac tamponade

Pneumomediastinum results from the abnormal presence of air within the mediastinum that may originate from a tear in the trachea, in a main-stem bronchus or in the esophagus, or from extension of subcutaneous emphysema (Table 2-10). The tracheal wall is identified because of air contrasting both the inside and outside of the tracheal rings. The major cranial vessels are clearly seen. The aorta and caudal portion of the esophagus are identified within the caudal mediastinum in some traumatized animals.

Mediastinal shift occurs with pulmonary injury or pleural lesions.

Table 2-10:
Radiographic signs of pneumomediastinum

1. better visualization of esophagus, trachea, and major vessels (lateral view) (Fig. 2-37)
2. pneumopericardium (both views)
3. visualization of a mediastinal mass
4. pneumoretroperitoneum (Fig. 2-37)

Damage to the heart and great vessels is uncommon, with traumatic injuries of the cardiovascular system seldom recognized radiographically. Comparison of the appearance of the heart on both orthogonal radiographic views is important in establishing the true anatomy of the heart in three dimensions. Configuration of the thorax greatly influences the appearance of the heart shadow. Shock in the traumatized animal causes hypovolemia and microcardia whereas hemopericardium causes cardiomegaly. The shape of the heart is altered by patient positioning (DV versus VD, and right versus left lateral). The heart shadow can be elevated from the sternum with pneumothorax.

Myocardial contusion is caused by impact to the heart and cannot be evaluated radiographically; however, it can cause bleeding with hemothorax, hemopericardium, and hemomediastinum that can be distinguished.

Hemothorax is the collection of blood in the pleural space and appears on both views radiographically as pleural effusion. Chylothorax may follow rupture of the thin-walled thoracic duct and denotes the presence of intestinal lymph in the pleural place. These are discussed under the heading of pleural fluid.

Mediastinal masses in traumatized animals are uncommon but may follow hemomediastinum. Granulomas may be secondary to infection and may mimic diaphragmatic hernia (Fig. 2-38). A more acute esophageal perforation causes a mediastinitis characterized by fluid accumulation within the mediastinum. In some animals, the cause of the esophageal rupture can be identified (Fig. 2-39). The most common cause of suspected mediastinal mass is deposition of fat due to obesity (Fig. 2-40).

Figure 2-1.
Normal lateral (A) and dorsoventral (B) thoracic radiographs .

It is important to evaluate the radiographs systematically by examining: (1) the periphery of the thorax, (2) the pleural space, (3) the lung parenchyma, and (4) the mediastinum.

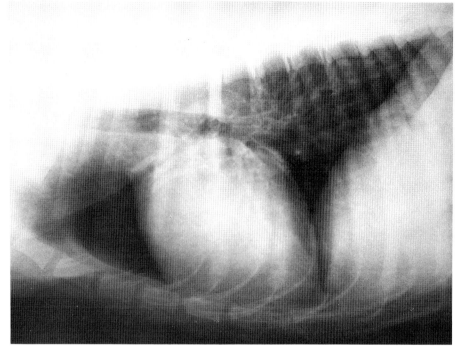

A

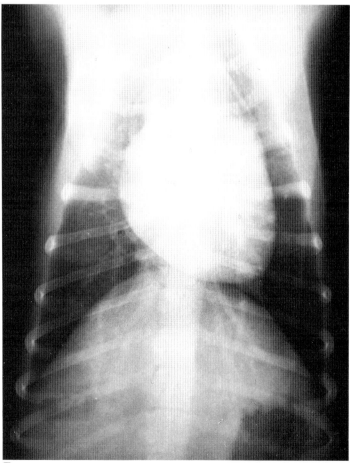

B

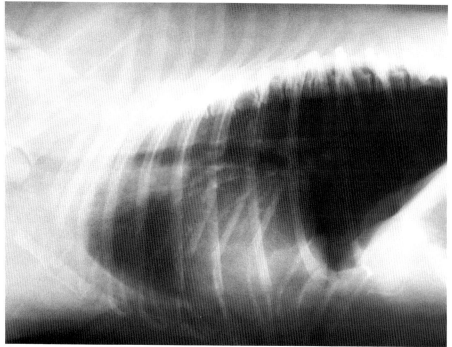

A

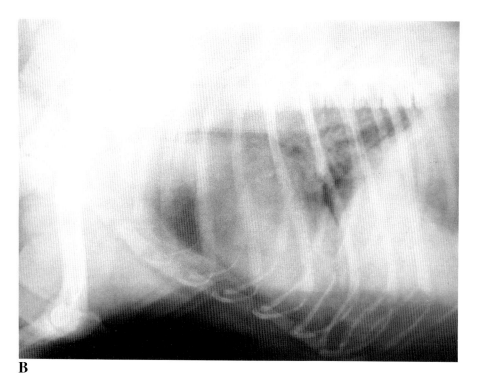

B

Figure 2-2.
Inspiratory (A) and expiratory (B) thoracic radiographs.
Note the difference in distance between the cardiac silhouette and diaphragm. Evaluation of the triangular area bounded cranially by the caudal portion of the cardiac silhouette, dorsally by the caudal vena cava, and caudally by the diaphragmatic shadow gives information of the degree of thoracic inspiration.

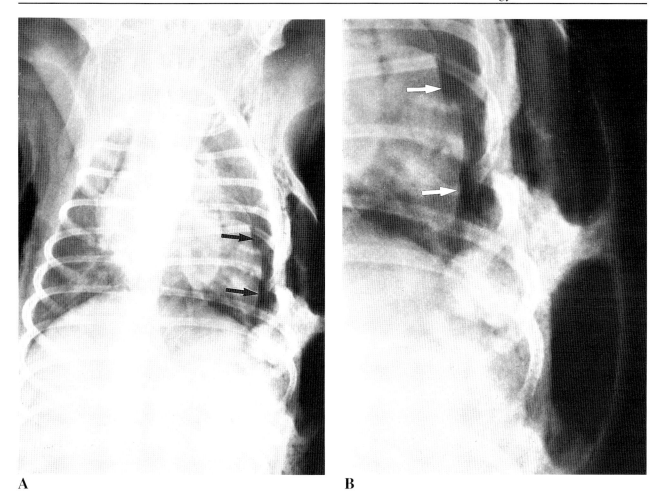

A

B

Figure 2-3.
Flail chest.
A 9-year-old Toy Poodle was bitten by a larger dog and was presented with clinical signs of dyspnea and a flail segment in the left thoracic wall. The dorsoventral thoracic radiographs proved to be helpful in the evaluation of the lesions. The sixth and seventh left ribs were fractured both dorsally and ventrally (at the costo-chondral junction). As a result, a flail segment was present. Under the skin, a large amount of air had collected. Inside the thoracic cavity, a unilateral pneumothorax with consolidation of the left lung lobes was visible (arrows). In addition, the ninth rib was fractured and the tenth rib was displaced. The right hemithorax seems to be undamaged, with only a minor amount of subcutaneous emphysema present.

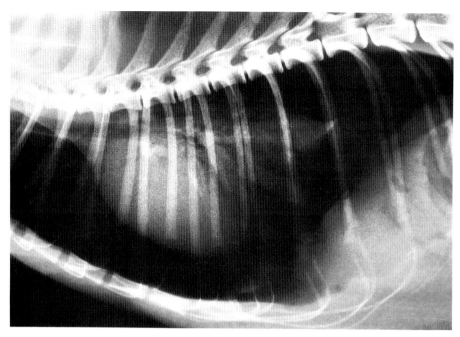

Figure 2-4.
Decreased radiographic density with thoracic trauma.
Severe pneumothorax with lung lobe atelectasis in a 1-year-old domestic short-haired cat results in overall decreased radiographic density (or increased radiolucency) of the thoracic image due to a large amount of free air in the pleural space.

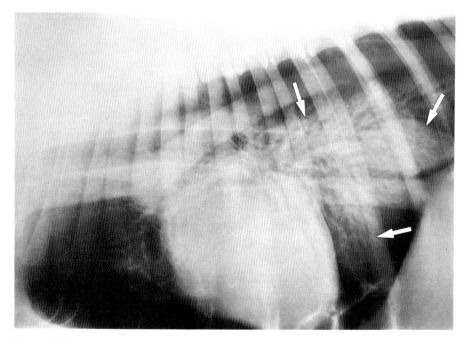

Figure 2-5.
Pneumothorax.
Following a collision with a car this 7-year-old German Shepherd Dog became very dyspneic. Thoracic radiographs revealed a bilateral pneumothorax with partial collapse of all lung lobes (arrows). Because no external thoracic wall lesions could be detected, pneumothorax was thought to be the result of intrinsic lung rupture.

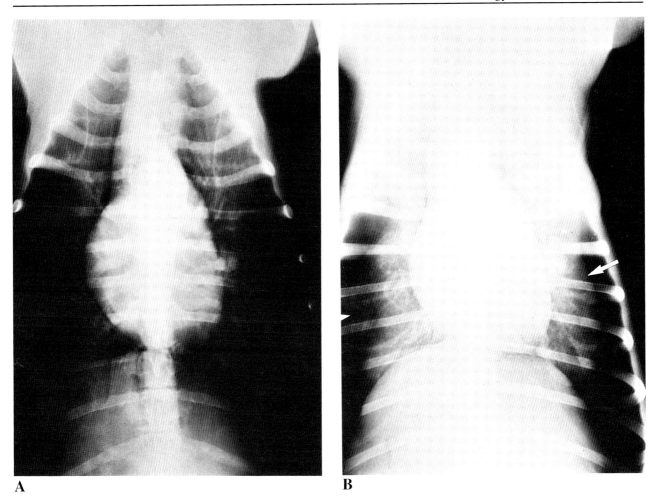

A   B

Figure 2-6.
Pneumothorax.
*In patients with pneumothorax, the routine exposure settings for thoracic radiographs results in "black-out" sections as a result of the increased amount of air that is present within the thorax (**A**). Using an underexposure technique (1/2 mAs setting), the borders of the recoiled lung lobes (arrows) are much easier to visualize (**B**). For evaluation of additional thoracic abnormalities, the routine radiographic technique is required.*

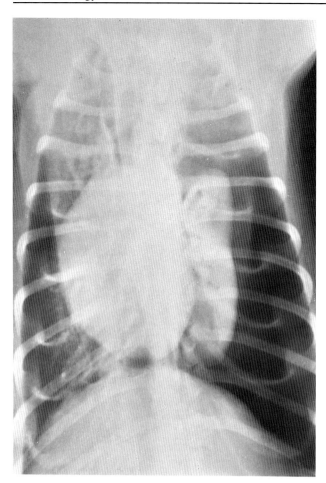

Figure 2-7.
Unilateral pneumothorax.
Spontaneous unilateral pneumothorax of the right hemithorax occurred in a 6-month-old Dachshund. The left lung lobes are completely collapsed and surrounded by a large amount of free pleural air that compresses and repositions the mediastinum slightly toward the right side. Also, the heart has moved to the right. All right lung lobes appear to inflate normally. Notice the shadow caused by the skin folds bilaterally and imagine how easy it would be to make the mistaken diagnosis of a pneumothorax.

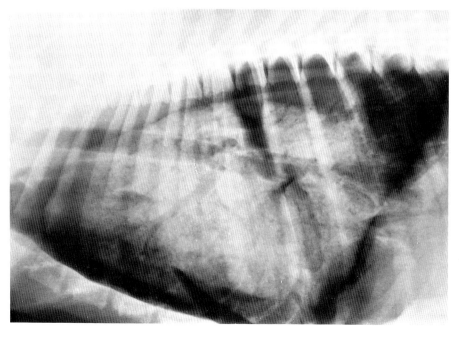

Figure 2-8.
Pneumothorax with pulmonary hemorrhage.
Several days after collision with a car, this 1-year-old Belgian Shepherd Dog became increasingly dyspneic. Thoracic radiographs revealed a moderate bilateral pneumothorax with partial lung lobe atelectasis. However, the lung lobes showed an unusual increased radiodensity and had air-bronchograms. These pulmonary changes are indicative of pulmonary hemorrhage in addition to pneumothorax-induced lung lobe collapse.

Figure 2-9.

Pneumothorax with diaphragmatic hernia.

This 4-year-old Weimaraner was very dyspneic after a traffic accident. Also, the abdominal cavity appeared to be empty on palpation. Radiographs revealed a severe pneumothorax with lung lobe atelectasis, but also the presence of an abnormal mass-lesion (arrows) in the ventral part of the thoracic cavity. The mass seemed to dislocate the heart in a dorso-cranial direction. The mass proved to be a part of the liver that had herniated through the diaphragmatic tear.

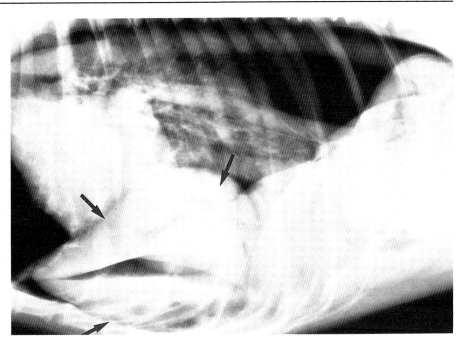

Figure 2-10.

Pseudo-pneumothorax.

Superimposition of skin folds (arrows) in a 9-year-old Scottish Sheepdog resemble a bilateral pneumothorax. Use of a bright spotlight device is sometimes necessary to enable the clinician to follow the pulmonary vessels and lung structures as they continue towards the periphery of the thoracic cavity, proving that the lungs fill the thoracic cavity completely and that there is no pneumothorax.

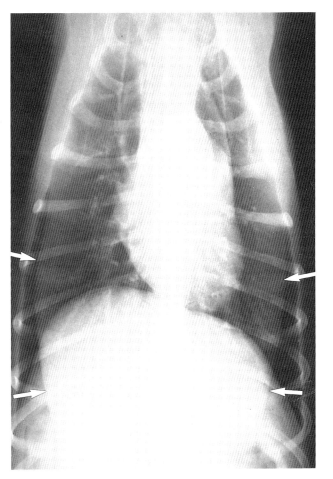

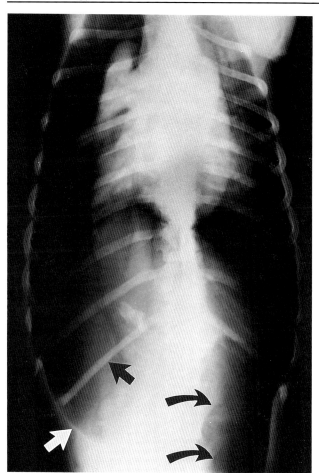

A

Figure 2-11.
Tension pneumothorax.
*Following trauma, a bilateral tension pneumothorax developed in a 1-year-old mixed breed dog resulting in increased dyspnea. The dorsoventral radiograph (**A**) offers a good impression of the caudal extension of the air-filled pleural space on the right side (straight arrows). On the left side, the presence of gas in the gastric fundus (curved arrows) mimics caudal extension of the pleural space. The right-sided lung lobes are completely collapsed and condensed while the left-sided lobes are still partially inflated. A second lateral radiograph (**B**) made with the dog in standing position using a horizontal beam projection demonstrates the presence of a large amount of free air in the dorsal region of the thoracic cavity delineating a flattened diaphragm, the aorta (curved arrows) and esophagus (straight arrows). In this position, the collapsed lung lobes are located ventrally around the cardiac shadow.*

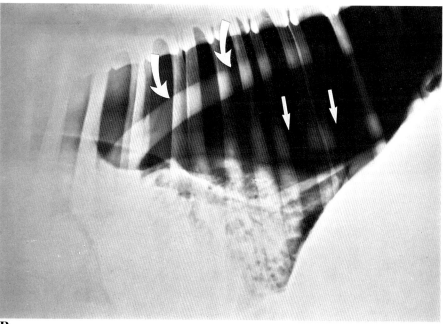

B

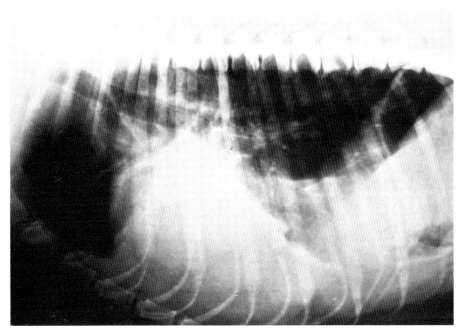

Figure 2-12.
Hemothorax.
A 3-year-old Cocker Spaniel had been hit by a car and was presented with paper-white mucous membranes. In addition to ruptures of the liver and spleen, the patient had a collection of free pleural fluid around the cardiac shadow that was visible radiographically. Post-mortem examination proved this to be due to pleural hemorrhage as a result of pericardial laceration and myocardial contusion.

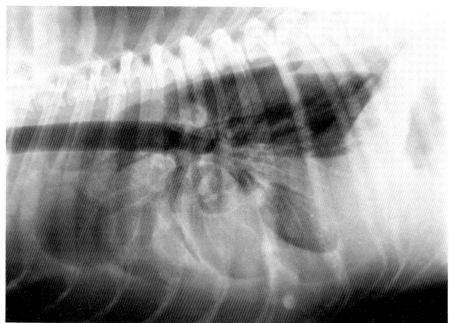

A

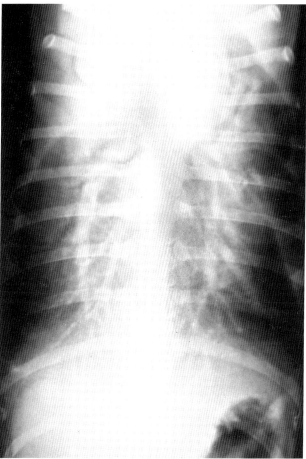

B

Figure 2-13.
Pleural effusion.
A post-traumatic liquothorax in a 7-year-old Bouvier (**A, B**) *offers all the characteristic radiographic signs of pleural effusion. Remember that it is impossible to distinguish the different causes of pleural fluid radiographically.*

Figure 2-14.
Diaphragmatic hernia.
In a traumatized 1-year-old Dachshund, the dorsoventral radiograph of the thorax presented an incomplete diaphragmatic silhouette due to rupture of the left hemidiaphragm and consequent intrathoracic displacement of abdominal viscera.

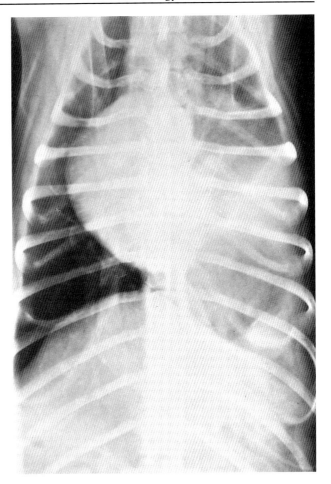

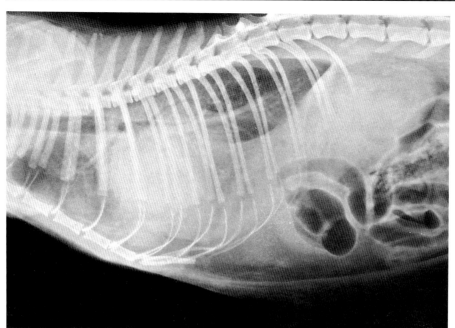

A

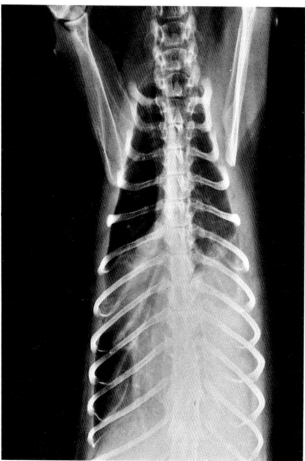

B

Figure 2-15.
Diaphragmatic hernia.
*The lateral radiograph (**A**) of this adult domestic short-haired cat reveals an incomplete diaphragmatic silhouette and obscured cardiac apex due to positive silhouetting of the heart with pleural fluid and displaced abdominal viscera. The ventrodorsal radiograph (**B**) that was made in an erect position with use of a horizontal beam projection presents an asymmetrical diaphragmatic outline, with displacement of the heart towards the right side.*

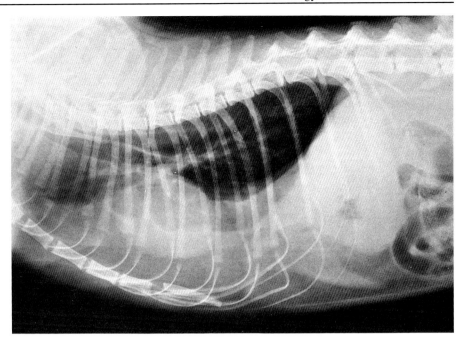

Figure 2-16.
Diaphragmatic hernia.
In a 5-year-old domestic short-haired cat with a traumatic diaphragmatic hernia, the cardiac apex is obscured by dislocated fat of the falciform fat triangle that has been displaced from its normal location intra-abdominally ventral to the liver.

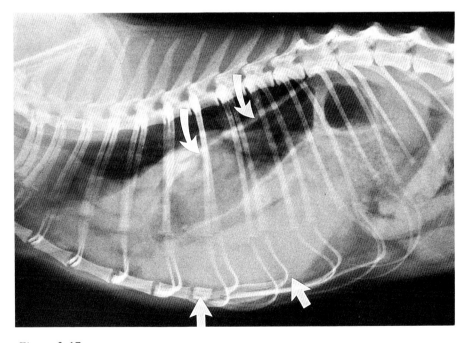

Figure 2-17.
Diaphragmatic hernia.
Following diaphragmatic rupture in a 1-year-old domestic short-haired cat, the liver (straight arrows) and gas-filled large bowel (curved arrows) are visible inside the thoracic cavity.

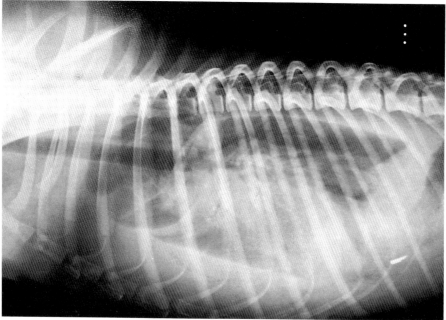

A

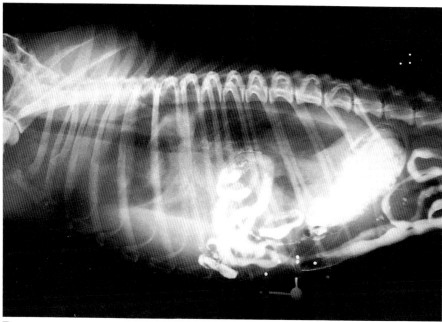

B

Figure 2-18.

Diaphragmatic hernia.

Routine non-contrast thoracic radiographs of a traumatized 5-year-old cross-breed dog confirmed the clinical diagnosis of pleural effusion (A). Due to the accumulation of fluid, the diaphragmatic silhouette is obscured and the possible presence of abdominal viscera concealed. There were no other signs of thoracic trauma. A barium swallow proved the presence of small bowel loops within the thoracic cavity (B). The position of the stomach is abnormal, with cranial displacement of the antrum and duodenum. The ventrally located soft tissue density proved to be the herniated liver.

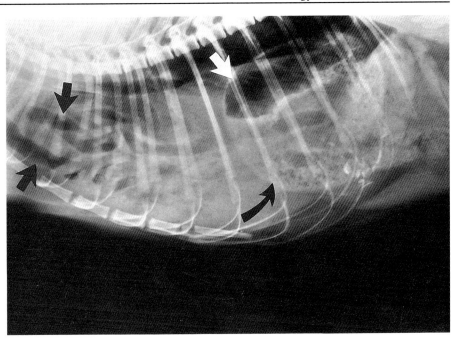

Figure 2-19.
Diaphragmatic hernia.
In an adult domestic short-haired cat, most of the intestinal loops are present inside the thoracic cavity. The gas-filled small intestinal loops are displaced cranially (straight arrows) while the feces-filled large bowel is located more caudally (curved arrow).

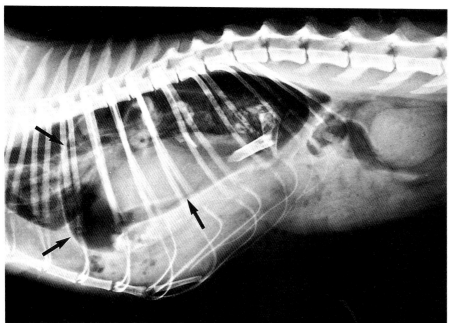

A

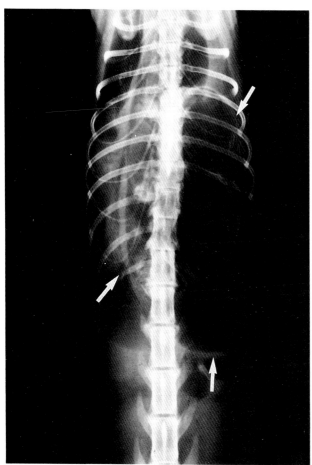

B

Figure 2-20.
Diaphragmatic hernia.
A 3-year-old domestic short-haired cat with known history of diaphragmatic hernia became suddenly severely dyspneic during the last 2 days before presentation. The lateral thoracic radiograph (A) reveals a largely distended, gas-filled stomach inside the thoracic cavity (arrows). The dorsoventral radiograph (B) shows displacement of the mediastinum and heart to the right side due to compression by the distended intrathoracic stomach (arrows).

Figure 2-21.
Diaphragmatic hernia.
This 1-year-old domestic short-haired cat with a diaphragmatic hernia has had repeated trauma. There are 6 recent rib fractures visible in the right thoracic wall. These fractures are at least 14 days old because of the periosteal callus that is already visible. An old healed rib fracture can be identified involving the ninth rib on the left side.

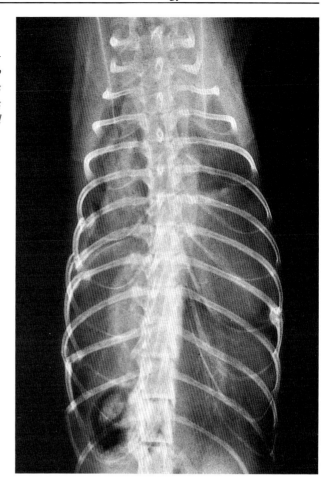

Figure 2-22.
Diaphragmatic hernia.
The abdominal cavity is nearly empty due to displacement of the abdominal viscera into the thoracic cavity following a traumatic diaphragmatic rupture in this 6-year-old domestic short-haired cat. Only the kidneys, urinary bladder and colon (arrows) are visible within the abdominal cavity.

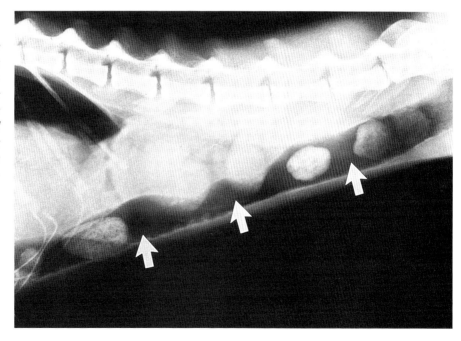

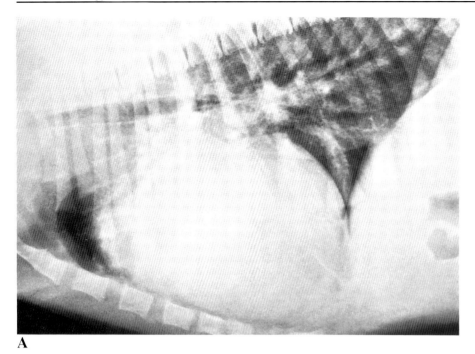

A

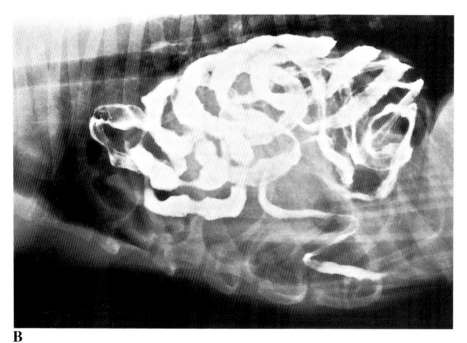

B

Figure 2-23.
Peritoneo-pericardial hernia.
On a non-contrast radiograph of a 3-month-old Deerhound, the cardiac shadow is larger than normal and positioned in close contact with the diaphragm (A). There are no radiographic signs of right-sided or left-sided cardiac failure. A barium study revealed the presence of small bowel loops inside the pericardial sac (B).

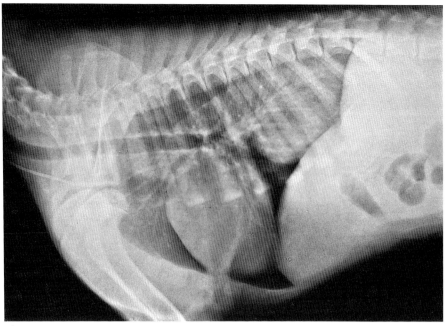

A

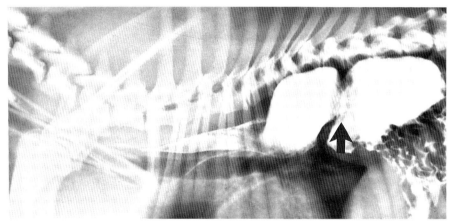

B

Figure 2-24.
Paraesophageal mediastinal hernia.
*In this 3-month-old Boxer puppy, a well-circumscribed soft tissue density was noted in the caudodorsal region of the non-contrast thoracic radiograph (**A**). In the cranial abdomen, a normal gastric shadow was not seen. An esophageal barium contrast examination revealed cranial displacement of the stomach through an enlarged diaphragmatic hiatus (**B**). The gastric cardia has an intrathoracic position (arrow) and the esophagus is abnormally dilated.*

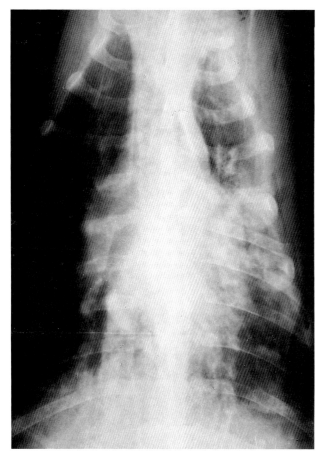

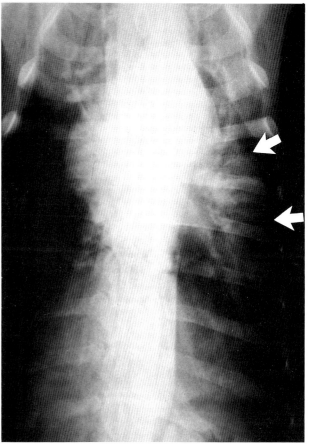

Figure 2-25.
Pulmonary contusion.
Following a crush injury to the left thoracic wall, thoracic radiographs of this 6-year-old German Shepherd Dog presented not only with fractures of the fifth and sixth left ribs, but also with an irregular, patchy, alveolar density pattern in the left lung lobes indicating pulmonary contusion.

Figure 2-26.
Pulmonary contusion and consolidation.
One day following blunt thoracic trauma, this 2-year-old cross-breed dog showed radiographic signs of pulmonary contusion and consolidation of the entire cardiac portion of the left cranial lung lobe (arrows). Note the air-bronchogram pattern. In addition, a small amount of free pleural fluid was present. No rib fractures were noted.

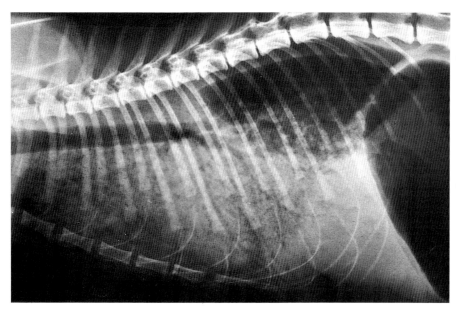

Figure 2-27.
Increased radiographic density following thoracic trauma.
Severe lung edema due to acute respiratory distress syndrome (ARDS) in a traumatized 1-year-old domestic short-haired cat resulted in increased pulmonary density radiographically. Notice the air-bronchograms in the affected lung lobes.

Figure 2-28.
Increased radiographic lung density following electric shock.
Severe lung edema in a perihilar location was present in a 8-month-old male kitten after it had bitten an electrical cord (110 Volt).

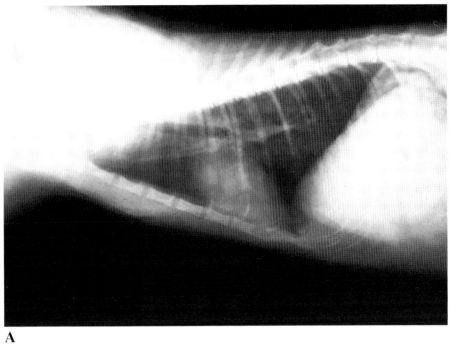

A

B

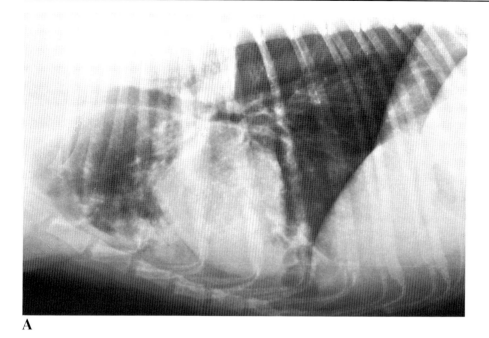

A

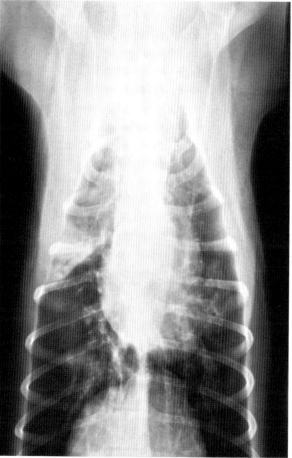

B

Figure 2-29.

Increased radiographic lung density following smoke inhalation.

*This 4-year-old, male Collie was rescued from a burning house, and brought into the clinic in comatose condition. The first radiographs that were taken several hours later (**A**, **B**) showed a lung pattern of mixed densities, with predominant peribronchial and alveolar infiltrates in the periphery of the ventral lung lobes and a consolidation in the caudodorsal area of the right cranial lung lobe. One week later (**C**), the mixed alveolar-peribronchial infiltrates were still visible, with increased impairment of the cranial lung lobes. The earlier dorsal consolidation had resolved partially. At 3 months (**D**), the lungs had regained their normal radiographic appearance, with minor pleural scarring as the only remnant of the earlier alveolar-peribronchial infiltrates.*

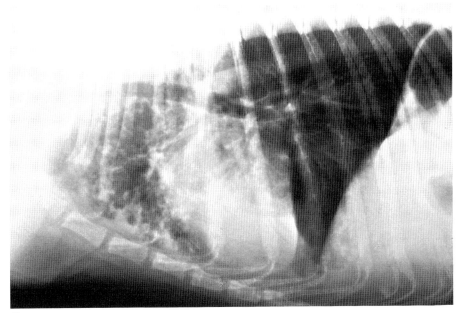

C

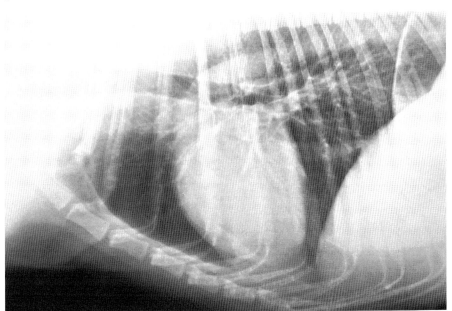

D

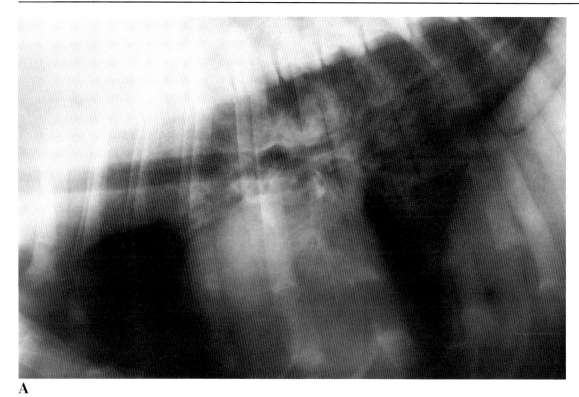

A

Figure 2-30.
Increased radiographic lung density following head trauma.
In a 1-year-old, female Great Dane that had sustained severe head trauma with fractures of the frontal bone, severe lung edema was present in a perihilar location. It is not possible to distinguish between pulmonary edema and pulmonary hemorrhage in this patient.

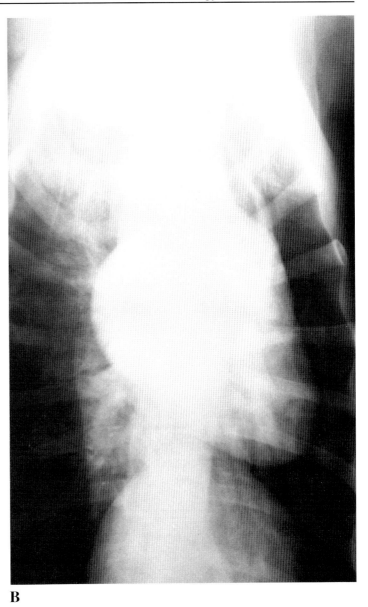

B

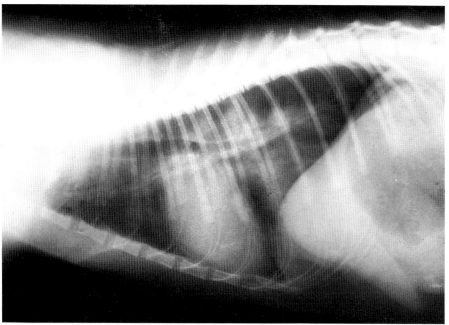

A

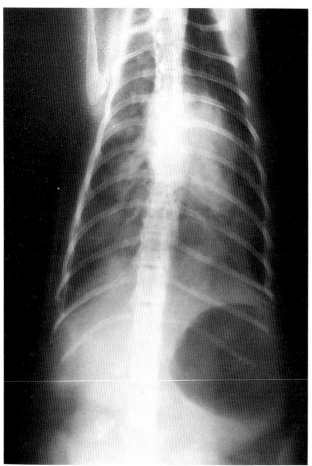

B

Figure 2-31.
Increased radiographic lung density following near-strangulation.

*Severe lung edema in the caudal lung lobes is noted in a 2-year-old, male cat (**A**, **B**) that had been caught in a garage door and suffered near-strangulation (asphyxiation). The same radiographic pattern was present in the lungs of an 8-month-old male Yorkshire Terrier that had been nearly strangulated by his collar when the leash had been trapped by a closed door (**C**, **D**).*

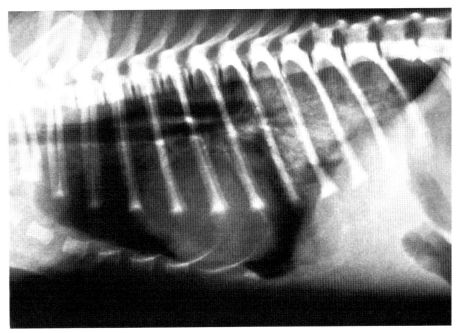

C

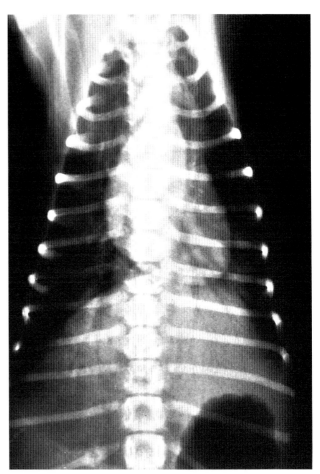

D

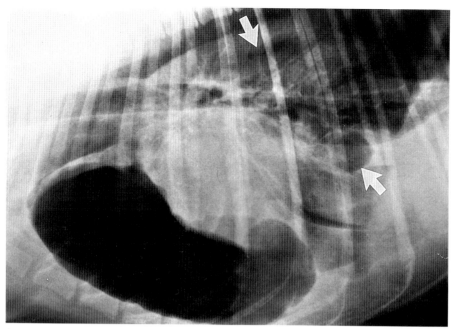

A

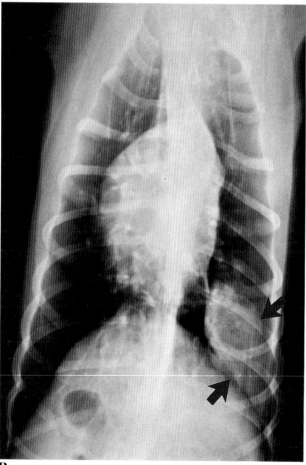

B

Figure 2-32.
Pulmonary hematoma.
Blunt thoracic trauma to a 2-year-old Scottish Sheepdog resulted in severe thoracic abnormalities and dyspnea. Thoracic radiographs revealed an extensive bilateral pneumothorax with moderate pleural effusion (**A**). The partially collapsed lung lobes contained several traumatic lung cysts (arrows). Following complete clinical recovery, control radiographs of the thorax were made 8 days later (**B**). The only remnant of the earlier thoracic abnormalities that was still visible on the radiographs was a localized soft tissue density within the ventral part of the left caudal lung lobe representing a pulmonary hematoma (arrows). After 3 months, only a small pulmonary scar could be detected radiographically at this site.

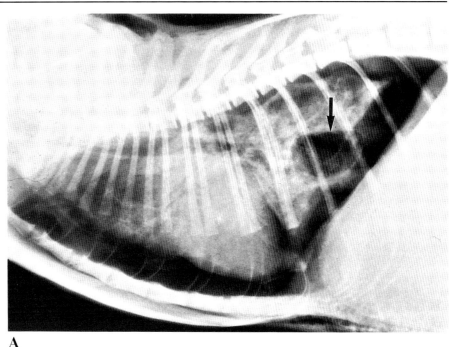

A

Figure 2-33.
Pulmonary bullae.

*Subcutaneous emphysema and pneumothorax are a frequent combination following thoracic trauma. Thoracic radiographs of a 6-month-old domestic short-haired cat that was bitten by a dog revealed free air within the pleural space (**A**) and accumulation of air in the subcutaneous tissues (**B**). The lungs were partially collapsed and presented with increased density due to lung contusion and hemorrhage. Several traumatic pulmonary cysts were also visible (arrows). The combination of subcutaneous emphysema and pneumothorax is a common sequel to perforating thoracic wall injuries. In these animals, the evaluation of additional pulmonary changes is very important.*

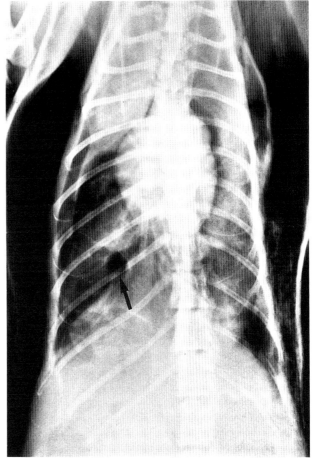

B

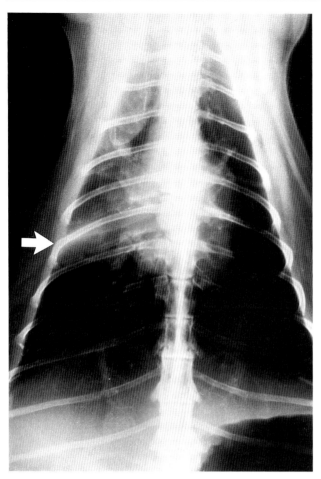

Figure 2-34.

Pulmonary thromboembolism.

Extensive pulmonary thrombosis in a 12-year-old domestic short-haired cat resulted in localized hyperlucency of several pulmonary regions due to interruption of normal vascular perfusion. This pattern may resemble pneumothorax radiographically. However, other signs of pneumothorax such as the recognition of recoiled lung lobe borders are not present. In this cat, the right cardiac lung lobe is consolidated as well (arrow).

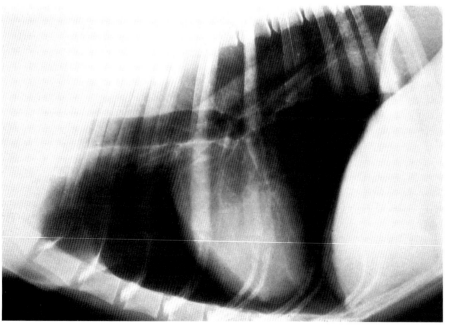

Figure 2-35.

Decreased radiographic density with thoracic trauma.

Hypovolemic shock in a 2-year-old German Shepherd Dog resulted in overall decreased radiographic density of the lungs due to underperfusion.

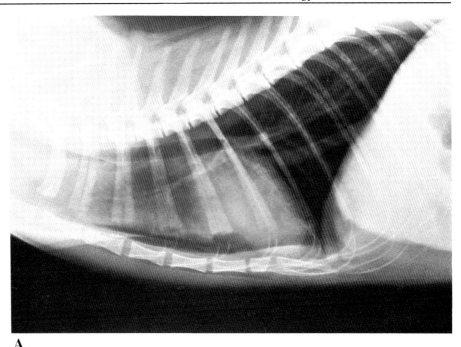

A

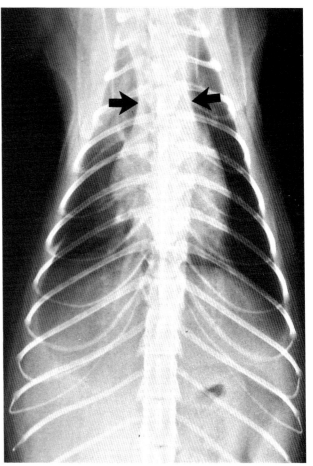

B

Figure 2-36.
Hemomediastinum.
*This 2-year-old domestic short-haired cat had survived a 10-meter fall without obvious clinical complaints. Thoracic radiographs revealed an increased density (**A**) and widening (**B**) of the precardiac mediastinum as a result of vascular rupture and consequent hemomediastinum. In cats, the precardiac mediastinum (arrows) should not be visible outside the contours of the thoracic vertebral column (in DV projection).*

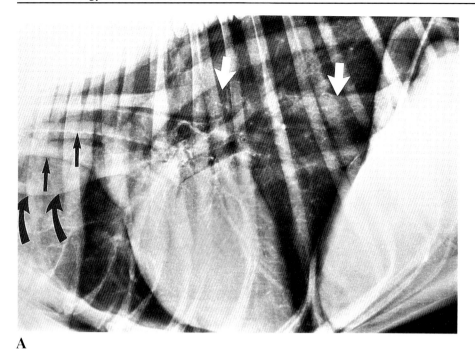

A

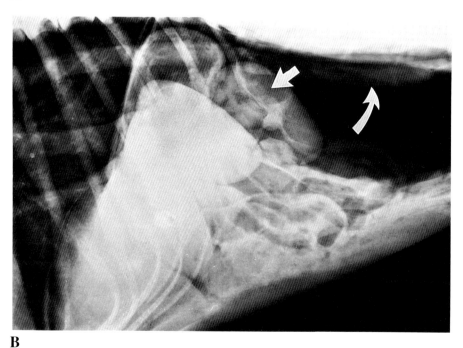

B

Figure 2-37.
Pneumomediastinum and pneumoretroperitoneum.
*Due to accumulation of air within the mediastinal space (pneumomediastinum) in an adult German Shepherd Dog, most of the mediastinal structures are sharply defined (**A**). The esophagus (thick arrows), aorta and aortic branches (thin arrows), and cranial vena cava (curved arrows) are all clearly visible, along with the tracheal walls and heart base. Due to migration of air through the esophageal and aortic hiatus of the diaphragm, air has also collected in the retroperitoneal space (pneumoretroperitoneum), resulting in clear definition of the retroperitoneal structures such as the kidneys (straight arrow) and abdominal aorta (curved arrow) (**B**).*

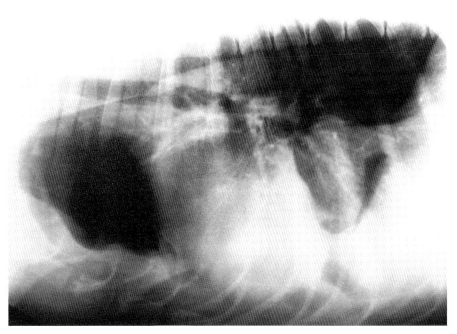

Figure 2-38.
Mediastinal mass.
In the caudoventral region of the thorax, a soft tissue mass partially obscures the out-line of the cardiac silhouette, caudal vena cava, and the diaphragm. No signs of free pleural fluid are noted. It is often difficult to differentiate radiographically between a subpleural or mediastinal mass and a traumatic diaphragmatic hernia. The mass le-sion in this 2-year-old Bouvier proved to be an actinomycotic granulomatous process involving the subpleural space, caudal mediastinum, pericardium and ventral dia-phragm.

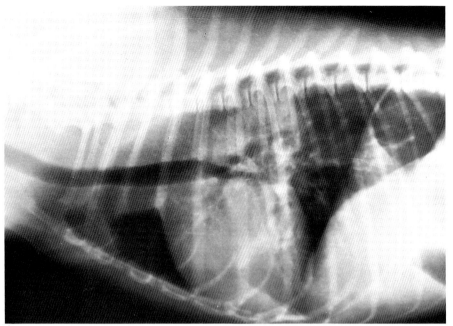

A

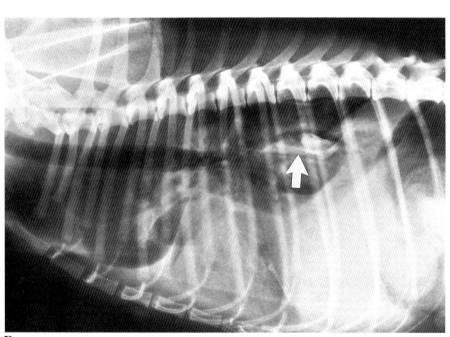

B

Figure 2-39.
Esophageal perforation.
Two dogs were presented following iatrogenic perforation of the esophagus in attempts to remove obstructing esophageal foreign bodies. One dog presented with radiographic signs of mediastinitis and mediastinal fluid accumulation (**A**), visible as increased density in the mediastinal area above the trachea and heart base. The other dog presented with signs of pleural effusion due to pleuritis (**B**). In the second patient, the foreign body was a piece of bone that remained lodged within the esophagus (arrow).

Figure 2-40.
Mediastinal fat or pseudo-liquothorax.
Abundant deposition of fat in the caudal mediastinal fissure (straight arrows) and precardiac mediastinum (curved arrows) of this adult cross-breed dog resembles the radiographic appearance of pleural effusion. The presence of pericardial fat (arrowheads) especially enlarges the silhouette of the right ventricular border in the dorsoventral projection.

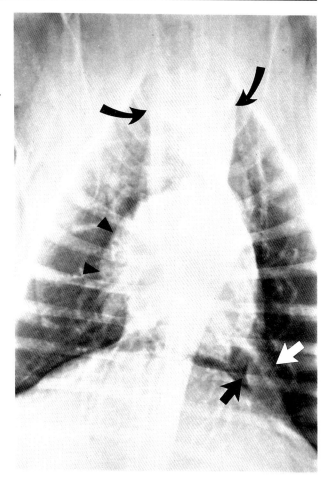

III. RADIOLOGY OF ABDOMINAL TRAUMA

1. Introduction

Trauma to the abdomen and the resulting injury to the intra-abdominal viscera is common. Causes of the trauma include traffic accidents, blunt trauma, perforating bite-wounds, penetrating trauma, gunshot injury, or the result of falling. Abdominal organs are seen to be more vulnerable than thoracic organs probably because they are not protected by a bony case. Early identification of the character of the injury influences how quickly treatment is undertaken and, as a result of this, the mortality rate. Iatrogenic trauma may result from perforations due to passage of a urinary catheter or following endoscopy, organ lacerations following paracentesis, inadvertent ligations during surgery, or post-surgical strictures or adhesions. This type of trauma is discussed in this text.

Abdominal trauma may include a number of specific injuries such as perforation and laceration of the body wall, laceration or rupture of organs, and avulsion of organs with resulting hemorrhage, bacterial or uremic peritonitis (Table 3-1).

It is important to consider that the trauma may not be limited, and injury to intrathoracic structures, diaphragm, vertebrae, and pelvis are often combined with injury to the abdominal organs.

The clinical signs of these animals vary from profound shock and/or dyspnea to lameness due to musculoskeletal injury. A careful physical examination may point out additional injuries to those clinically apparent.

Radiographic evaluation of abdominal radiographs of a traumatized animal must be performed in a systematic manner, including all anatomic structures. Peripheral soft tissues, surrounding bony structures, retroperitoneal space, peritoneal cavity, solid abdominal organs, and hollow vis-

Table 3-1:
Specific abdominal injuries secondary to trauma

1. body wall – laceration, perforation, herniation
2. liver – rupture, subcapsular hemorrhage, herniation, lobe avulsion
3. gall bladder – rupture, avulsion
4. spleen – torsion, subcapsular hemorrhage, herniation, rupture
5. pancreas – rupture
6. stomach – herniation, rupture, volvulus
7. bowel – mesenteric torsion/volvulus, perforation/rupture, infarction
8. kidney – subcapsular hemorrhage, rupture, avulsion, acute hydronephrosis
9. ureter – rupture, acute hydroureter, avulsion
10. urinary bladder – rupture, intramural hemorrhage, avulsion, herniation
11. urethra – rupture/tear
12. prostate gland – herniation
13. mesentery – tear, herniation

cera must be included. Injuries of this type present several unique diagnostic patterns and deserve separate consideration from the standpoint of diagnostic radiology in general.

2. Radiographic Changes due to Abdominal Trauma

2.1. Peripheral soft tissue trauma

The abdominal wall is identified radiographically due to the contrasting effects of the peritoneal fat and the fat tissue between the muscle layers. A radiographic diagnosis of abdominal wall injury is made when the normal structures of the lateral or ventral abdominal wall are not easily identified because the contrasting radiolucent fat lines are lost due to hemorrhage or edema. It is usually necessary to use a bright light to evaluate the character of the abdominal wall. Together with the loss of these linear fat shadows, it is possible that free gas shadows are present within the layers of the abdominal wall, when the original trauma has broken the skin and, as a result, subcutaneous emphysema is present.

If gas- or ingesta-filled bowel loops are herniated, their identification is relatively easy to make on the radiograph regardless of the direction of the herniation. A major form of peripheral soft tissue trauma is herniation with displacement of solid abdominal viscera outside the abdominal cavity through a diaphragmatic, paracostal, inguinal, perineal, ventral, or umbilical tear or rupture. If the liver or spleen are herniated, the ability to identify these structures is dependent on the surrounding environment. If the spleen is paracostal and surrounded by contrasting fat, it is visible. If the liver is intrathoracic and surrounded by pleural fluid, it is not possible to identify this structure radiographically. Often, soft tissue swellings suggest the possibility of hernia, but need to be differentiated from hematomas, seromas, or simply non-contained hemorrhage and/or edema. The use of orally administered contrast agents assists in the identification of herniated bowel loops, while the use of intravenously injected contrast agents assists in localization of a herniated urinary bladder. Radiographic signs of peripheral soft tissue trauma are listed in Table 3-2.

Table 3-2:
Radiographic signs of peripheral soft tissue trauma

1. obscured diaphragmatic outline (see chapter 2)
2. loss of identification of separate layers of abdominal wall (Fig. 3-1)
3. malpositioned bowel loops (Figs. 3-1, 3-2)
4. malpositioned solid organs
5. herniated viscera (Fig. 3-1)
6. subcutaneous emphysema (Figs. 3-1, 3-2)
7. rigid abdominal wall due to peritoneal irritation

2.2. Fractures

Fractures of the surrounding bony structures may suggest trauma to adjacent abdominal viscera (Table 3-3). The animal with a rupture of the urinary bladder or urethra should be carefully evaluated for pelvic or lumbosacral fracture/luxation. Fracture/luxations of the vertebrae are often seen in conjunction with abdominal injury and are overlooked because they may not be causing obvious neurologic signs.

Table 3-3:
Radiographic signs of fractures associated with abdominal trauma

1. classic appearance of fractured tubular bones with displacement of fragments
2. vertebral compression fractures with shortening of vertebral segments
3. rib fractures with minimal fragment displacement
4. multiple pelvic fractures (Fig. 3-2)
5. sacroiliac luxations

2.3. Peritoneal fluid

There are many causes of peritoneal fluid. It may be hemorrhagic and follow laceration or crushing of the liver, spleen, pancreas, or kidneys or rupture of an abdominal vessel. It may also be septic as the result of rupture of a hollow viscus. The peritoneal fluid is rarely caused by peritoneal irritation due to rupture of the gall bladder or pancreas. Peritonitis may be caused by the intra-abdominal presence of urine following rupture of the bladder or injury to the urethra or ureter at the bladder neck. An additional cause of peritoneal fluid results from volvulus, torsion, or incarceration of bowel with resulting passive congestion. It is usually not possible to determine the character of the peritoneal fluid from the radiograph, although certain generalizations can be made. The greater the quantity of fluid, the more likely it is due to effusion or urine. The more focal, the greater the possibility that the fluid is septic or hemorrhagic. Paracentesis is necessary to make a determination of its character.

Detection of peritoneal fluid on radiographs is sometimes difficult. It depends on the pattern of distribution throughout the abdominal cavity and its volume. If there is a large quantity of fluid distributed throughout the abdominal cavity, the radiograph will show abdominal distension and marked loss of intra-abdominal contrast. This may result in inability to identify the serosal surface of bowel loops and other abdominal viscera, as the bladder, liver, spleen, and abdominal wall. As a result it is impossible to identify these normally visible structures. In this case, there is little value in using positional radiographic techniques since it is not possible to move the fluid to a specific portion of the abdomen to assist in determining its origin.

If the volume of fluid is small or localized, radiographic diagnosis is much more difficult because of the smaller size of the abnormality. This diagnostic problem may occur with suspected pancreatic injury, where the resulting pancreatitis/peritonitis is localized, or with focal injury to the bowel with a resulting localized septic peritonitis. Positional films or compression studies may be helpful in such cases when trying to move overlying abdominal structures away from the site of localized peritoneal fluid collection (Table 3-4).

Table 3-4:
Radiographic signs of peritoneal fluid

1. increased density within the peritoneal space (Figs. 3-3, 3-4, 3-5, 3-6, 3-7)
2. non-visualization of the liver and/or spleen (Fig. 3-3, 3-4, 3-5, 3-6, 3-7)
3. non-visualization of the bladder (Fig. 3-7)
4. loss of serosal surface of the bowel (Figs. 3-3, 3-5, 3-7)
5. "floating" of bowel loops (Figs. 3-3, 3-6)
6. distended abdomen (Fig. 3-7)
7. non-visualization of abdominal wall (Fig. 3-7)

In patients that fail to recover from trauma in an expected manner, re-evaluation of the peritoneal space is indicated since it is possible that abdominal hemorrhage may not become visible until hours after the trauma when blood volume has been restored and blood pressure has returned to normal. Likewise, peritonitis may not be evident on early radiographs.

2.4. Retroperitoneal fluid

If the fluid is blood or urine and comes from an injured kidney or ureter, it often remains retroperitoneally and is identified radiographically by a large fluid-dense mass in a paravertebral location (Table 3-5). The accumulated fluid makes it impossible to identify the renal shadows because of positive silhouetting with these structures. The descending colon and rectum may be displaced ventrally. Vertebral fractures may be associated with the injury that causes the collection of retroperitoneal fluid. It is also possible that fluid accumulates within the retroperitoneal spaces of the pelvic cavity due to hemorrhage secondary to pelvic fractures or due to accumulation of urine following a bladder

Table 3-5:
Radiographic signs of retroperitoneal fluid

1. increased density of retroperitoneal space (Fig. 3-8)
2. non-visualization of kidneys (Fig. 3-8)
3. displacement of kidneys (Fig. 3-8)
4. asymmetry of renal size
5. enlarged kidney(s)
6. ventral displacement of descending colon and rectum (Fig. 3-8)
7. associated vertebral fractures
8. associated pelvic fractures (Fig. 3-8)

neck rupture or leakage from a retroflexed bladder.

2.5. Peritoneal air

The presence of peritoneal air follows perforation or rupture of a hollow viscus or a perforating wound through the abdominal wall. Small amounts of air are difficult to diagnose radiographically since the air remains in small pockets, trapped in the mesenteric folds. Because most abdominal radiographs are made with the patient recumbent, air bubbles are distributed over a large portion of the abdomen and are not seen tangentially in one large pocket. However, it helps to keep the animal in the same position on the radiographic table for 5-10 minutes, allowing the small air bubbles to collect into larger gas pockets. If a larger amount of air is present, it accumulates at the highest point of the abdominal cavity. When the radiograph is made in left lateral recumbency, the liver will be outlined. At the same time, both sides of the diaphragm become visible due to the contrasting effects of the pulmonary air cranially and the free peritoneal air caudally. On the dorsoventral view, the air accumulates around the kidneys. As a result, they are more easily visualized. This may be difficult to understand since the air is peritoneal and the kidneys are retroperitoneal; however, the kidneys are freely movable and fall ventrally so that peritoneal air contrasts sharply with the dense kidneys. Clear identification of the serosal surfaces of a bowel loop also indicates that peritoneal air is present. Sometimes, a "tramline-like" configuration exists when the walls of a gas-filled intestinal loop are contrasted on both sides, internally by the intestinal gas and externally by the peritoneal gas.

The easiest method of confirming the suspected presence of peritoneal air is to perform a radiographic study using a horizontal X-ray beam. By positioning the animal on the X-ray table for 10-15 minutes prior to making the exposure, the air col-

Table 3-6:
Radiographic signs of peritoneal air

1. air visible between liver and diaphragm (Fig. 3-9)
2. better visualization of the kidneys on DV view
3. visualization of serosal surface of the bowel
4. triangular shaped air pockets between bowel loops (Fig. 3-9)
5. air visualized using horizontal beam (Fig. 3-10)

lects in the uppermost portion of the abdominal cavity and creates a pocket that is more easily identified beneath the abdominal wall. Using left lateral positioning of the animal permits the gas to collect between the right diaphragmatic crus and the liver, and here it is most readily visible because it is identified away from the gas-filled bowel (Table 3-6).

It is important to remember that abdominal air is present for a period of several days to several weeks following laparotomy, abdominal paracentesis, or use of pneumoperitoneography as a diagnostic technique.

2.6. Peritoneal ingesta/feces
The detection of free ingesta or feces in the peritoneal cavity implies very severe stomach and/or bowel injury in an animal that will probably not survive the trauma. Still, it should be considered as an explanation of an unusual pattern of abdominal densities. The original injury may also cause free air to enter the peritoneal cavity thus confirming rupture of a hollow viscus.

2.7. Organ enlargement
Enlargement of abdominal organs may be due to subcapsular or encapsulated hemorrhage. This may occur following hepatic, splenic, or renal injury. Since the fluid is contained, the border of the organ remains visible on the radiograph but the organ itself appears larger or with a different shape or contour than usual (Figs. 3-11, 3-12).

2.8. Combination of patterns
Any of the patterns described above can be seen in combination with any other pattern. A herniated spleen with subcapsular hemorrhage and peritoneal bleeding combines radiographic changes in location and borderline of the organ with a change of the peritoneal cavity due to the presence of free fluid.

3. Use of Contrast Studies in the Traumatized Abdomen

3.1. Urinary tract trauma
Traumatic lesions of the urinary tract are frequent. In addition to non-contrast radiography, excretory urography and retrograde urethro-cystography can be very helpful diagnostic techniques. Excretory urography is the most easily performed study since the trauma patient probably has a venous catheter in place because of the requirement for fluid therapy. Therefore, injection of a positive-contrast urographic contrast agent in an amount of 1-2 ml/kg bw. can be conveniently performed. Radiographs made at 5 to 10 minutes after injection normally show bilateral function of both kidneys. In abnormal circumstances, one or both kidneys may fail to excrete the contrast agent because of renal artery thrombosis or renal artery tear. Enlarged renal shadows may be due to hydronephrosis resulting from ureteral rupture or obstruction. Contrast medium may accumulate within the renal subcapsular space indicating renal laceration. The contrast may leak into the retroperitoneal space indicating renal laceration or into the peritoneal space when the kidney is lacerated and the peri-

toneum torn. Later studies may show leakage of contrast from a torn ureter, and subsequent studies will reveal the position of the bladder and the character of the bladder wall (Table 3-7).

If it is possible to catheterize the urinary bladder in a retrograde direction, the location of the bladder and the status of the bladder wall can be determined. By repositioning the catheter tip more distally within the urethra, it is possible to ascertain the integrity of the urethral wall (Table 3-8).

Table 3-7:
Radiographic signs of urinary tract trauma following excretory urography

1. extravasation of contrast medium into retroperitoneal space (Figs. 3-13, 3-14)
2. extravasation of contrast medium into renal subcapsular space
3. extravasation of contrast medium into peritoneal space (Fig. 3-14)
4. failure of normal renal opacification/excretion (Fig. 3-13)
5. hydronephrosis
6. hydroureter
7. failure to visualize bladder (Fig. 3-15)

Table 3-8:
Radiographic signs of urinary tract trauma following retrograde urethro-cystography
1. extravasation of contrast medium into peritoneal space (Figs. 3-16 , 3-17, 3-18)
2. extravasation of contrast medium into retroperitoneal (intrapelvic) space (Fig. 3-19)
3. extravasation of contrast medium into the periurethral space (Fig. 3-19)
4. bladder displacement (Fig. 3-20)
5. hydroureter
6. pelvic fractures (Fig. 3-16)

3.2. Gastrointestinal tract trauma
Traumatic lesions of the gastrointestinal tract are infrequent and are generally identified through evaluation of non-contrast radiographs. Occasionally, administration of an oral contrast agent is helpful in the detection of lesions involving a part of the gastrointestinal tract. These contrast studies are usually performed by oral administration of a barium sulfate suspension. Radiographs are made at varying time intervals following administration of the contrast medium dependent on the information to be gained (Table 3-9).

Often the important radiographic finding is the location of the hollow viscus. Displacement of a part of the gastrointestinal tract is common in hernias and this is readily determined by identifying the positive-contrast medium within the stomach or small bowel. In most animals, traumatic peritonitis causes a marked difference in the appearance of the bowel loop(s). In animals in which there is rupture of the wall of stomach or bowel, it is possible that the tear is large enough to identify the extravasation of the barium. Today, it is advisable not to use barium suspensions in animals in which gastrointestinal perforation is suspected since peritoneal spillage of the barium suspension will result in granulomatous and adhesive peritonitis. With these animals, if a contrast investigation is necessary at all, it is advisable to use one of the recently developed water-soluble contrast agents such as iopamidol or iohexol.

Table 3-9:
Radiographic signs of gastrointestinal trauma following orally administered barium contrast medium

1. displacement of stomach or small bowel
2. abnormal appearance of bowel (Fig. 3-21)
3. extravasation of contrast medium into peritoneal space
4. extravasation of contrast medium into subcutaneous space

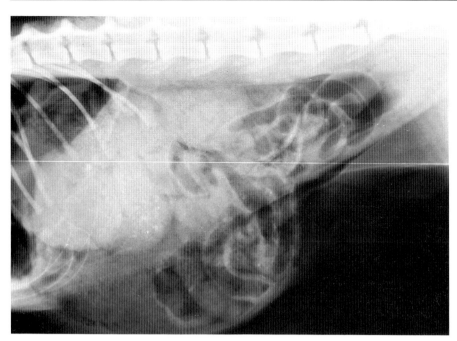

Figure 3-1.
Complicated ventral hernia.
This 1-year-old domestic short-haired cat came home with a large soft tissue swelling extending from the ventral abdominal wall. Radiographs revealed the real nature and contents of the swelling and showed it to be a ventral hernia containing dislocated falci-form fat and several small bowel loops. In addition, many free small gas bubbles are visible in the surrounding soft tissues. Surgery revealed perforation of one of the herniated small intestinal loops. Notice that all small bowel loops are dilated due to traumatic paralytic ileus.

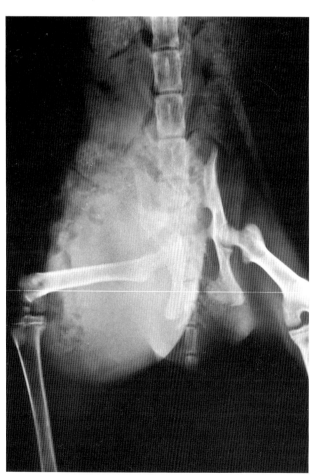

Figure 3-2.
Inguinal hernia.
Following a traffic accident, this 7-month-old domestic short-haired cat presented with multiple pelvic fractures and a right-sided inguinal hernia containing bowel loops and a large hematoma.

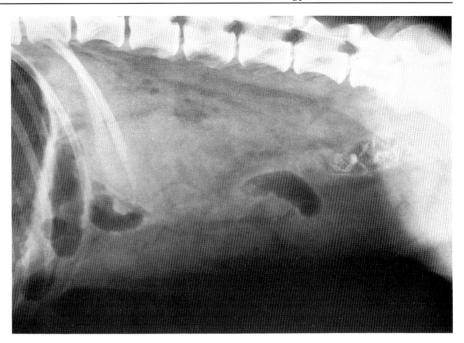

Figure 3-3.
Hemoperitoneum following splenic rupture.
Abdominal radiographs of a lethargic 2-year-old German Shepherd Dog revealed generalized increased density with loss of detail of the abdominal cavity. These radiographic changes are highly indicative of intraperitoneal fluid accumulation. Surgery proved the presence of hemoperitoneum due to splenic rupture.

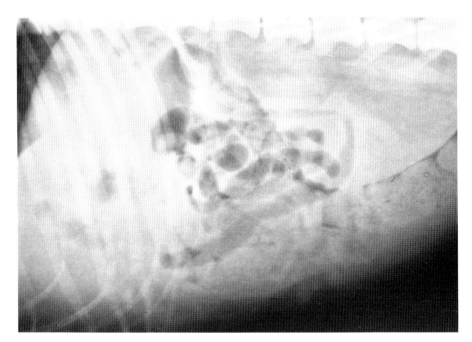

Figure 3-4.
Hydroperitoneum due to gall-bladder rupture.
The generalized increased density pattern that is visible on the abdominal radiograph of a traumatized 3-year-old Labrador Retriever was due to a perforated gall-bladder. Trauma occurred one week earlier.

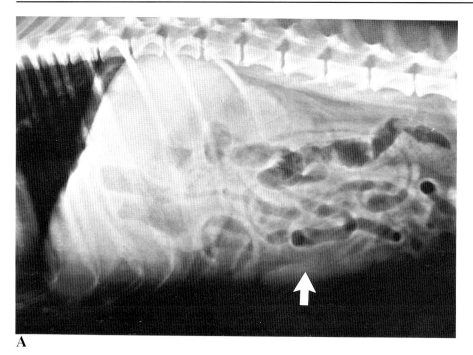

A

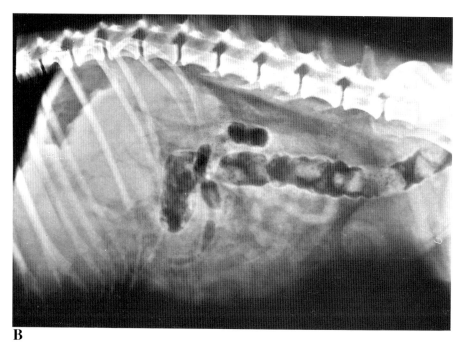

B

Figure 3-5.

Traumatic mesenteric hemorrhage.

*A 9-year-old Poodle was presented with clinical signs of abdominal pain following a kick in the abdomen by an unfriendly neighbour. The first radiograph was made 1 hour after the accident and did not reveal any radiographic abnormalities. The liver, spleen (arrow), kidneys, and small bowel loops were outlined in normal detail (**A**). The second radiograph was made 4 hours after the accident and showed loss of detail and increased density in the ventral abdomen (**B**). Notice that the spleen is no longer visible. Surgery revealed abdominal hemorrhage due to a mesenteric tear.*

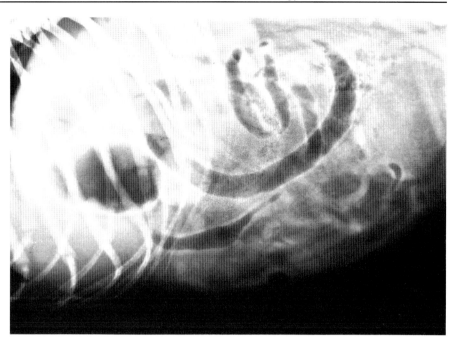

Figure 3-6.
Traumatic peritonitis.
Following a traffic accident, this 14-year-old cross-breed dog became lethargic and presented with a very rigid abdomen. The abdominal radiograph showed loss of detail in the mid-abdomen with dilatation of several small intestinal loops in the same region. These are radiographic signs of traumatic peritonitis. Surgery proved a pre-perforative peritonitis due to small bowel wall contusion.

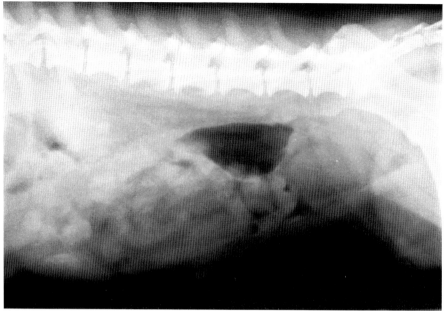

A

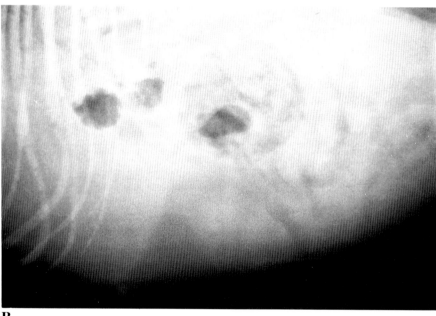

B

Figure 3-7.
Delayed peritoneal fluid accumulation.
*Directly following blunt abdominal trauma, a 4-year-old Dachshund presented at the clinic with no abnormal physical signs or radiographic changes (**A**). Five days later, the dog returned with a severely distended abdomen due to peritoneal collection of a large amount of fluid (**B**). Paracentesis was performed and a large amount of urine was removed. During surgery, a large bruise was identified on the wall of the urinary bladder through which the urine was leaking diffusely.*

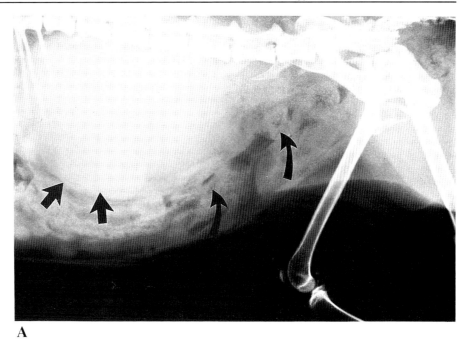

A

Figure 3-8.
Retroperitoneal hematoma.
A 3-year-old domestic short-haired cat was presented 10 days after a traffic accident with right-sided abdominal distension and abnormal motion of the hind legs. Lateral abdominal radiographs (A) revealed a large soft tissue density in the right retroperitoneal space that displaced the right kidney (straight arrows) and colon (curved arrows) ventrally. On the ventrodorsal projection (B), only the left kidney was visible while the unilateral location of the mass was obvious. The soft tissue mass proved to be a large retroperitoneal hematoma. Notice the multiple pelvic fractures and ileo-sacral luxation.

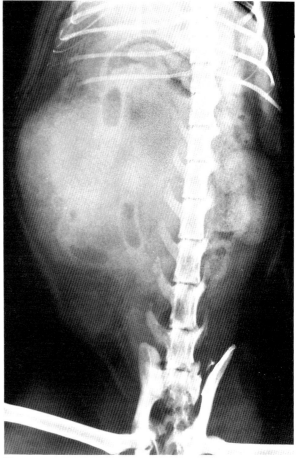

B

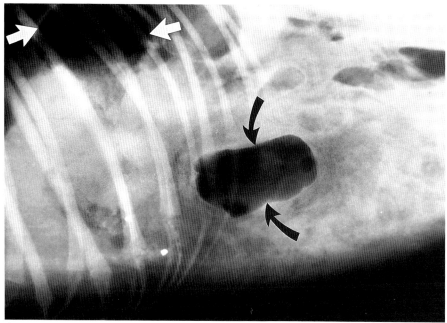

A

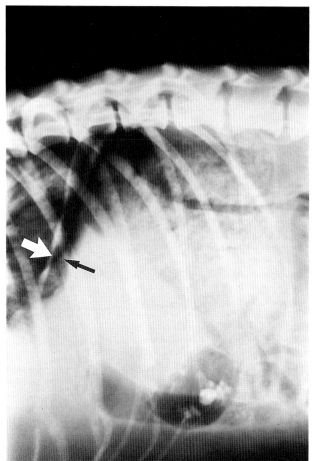

B

Figure 3-9.

Free peritoneal gas due to gastrointestinal perforation.

*Abdominal pain and distension were the main clinical signs in an 11-year-old Afghan Hound that was kicked by a horse, 3 days earlier. An abdominal radiograph (**A**) revealed increased abdominal density due to free peritoneal fluid and pockets of free gas indicating intra-abdominal perforation (no external lesions present). Free gas accentuates the radiographic outline of the wall of the gastric fundus (straight arrows) while a second loculated gas-pocket is visible in the mid-abdominal region (curved arrows).*

*In a second dog (**B**), a 7-year-old cross-breed with the same clinical complaints, free peritoneal gas was found at the highest point of the abdominal cavity between the diaphragm and the liver. With the patient in left lateral recumbency, this is the area where smaller amounts of free peritoneal gas collect producing a radiolucent separation between the right diaphragmatic crus (thick arrow) and the liver (thin arrow). Intragastric food and gas partially superimpose this radiographic finding.*

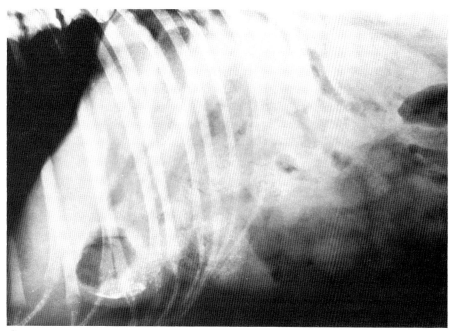

A

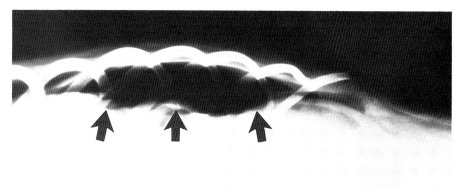

B

Figure 3-10.
Free peritoneal gas seen using a horizontal beam projection.
*Following blunt abdominal trauma, abdominal radiographs of an adult Irish Setter showed a questionable abdominal picture with suspicion of free peritoneal gas (**A**). To confirm the finding, a horizontal beam projection was made with the patient in left lateral recumbency (**B**). Free peritoneal gas collected at the highest point beneath the rib cage (arrows).*

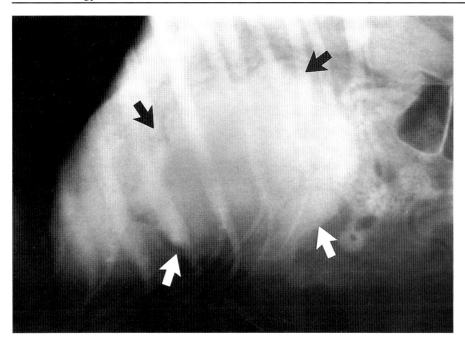

Figure 3-11.
Encapsulated hemorrhage of liver.
An 11-year-old Doberman Pinscher (Doberman) was kicked by a horse. At clinical presentation, no external traumatic lesions were noticed. However, the dog's clinical situation deteriorated quickly. Abdominal radiographs presented an irregular soft tissue mass that seemed to extend from the liver (arrows). Emergency surgery revealed a large subcapsular hematoma of the liver that ruptured during palpation.

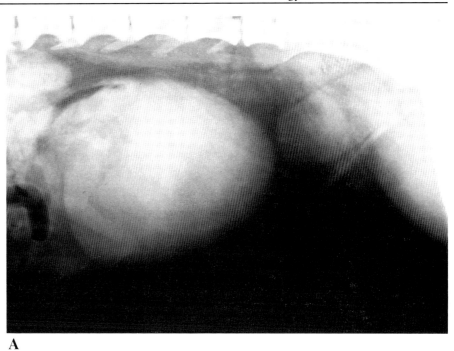

A

Figure 3-12.
Subcapsular splenic hematoma.
The well-circumscribed soft tissue mass in the mid-abdomen of this 9-year-old cross-breed dog was due to a subcapsular hematoma of the spleen following a traffic accident. Splenic hematomas can become large and occupy different regions of the abdominal cavity depending upon what part of the spleen is lacerated.

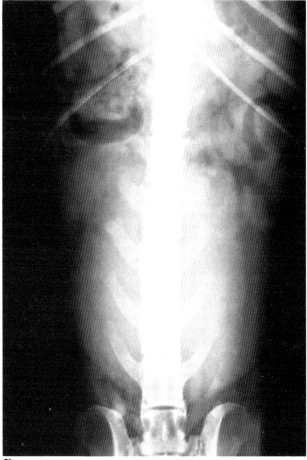

B

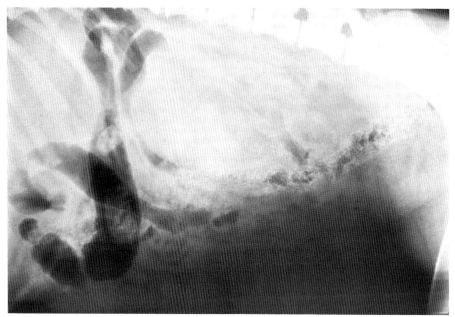

A

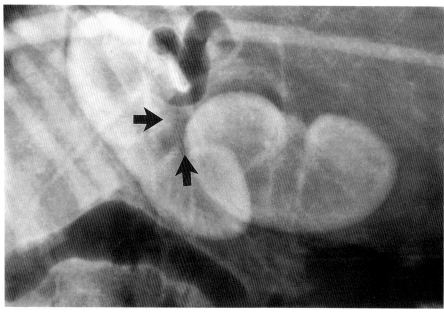

B

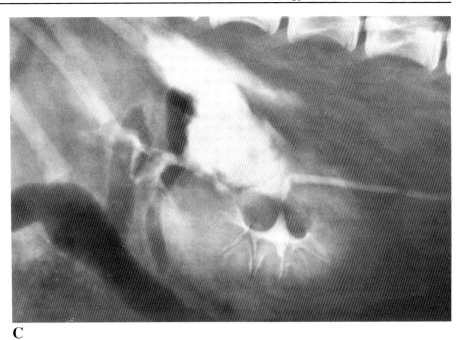

C

Figure 3-13.
Retroperitoneal urinoma due to kidney trauma.
*An 8-month-old Hovawarth became severely depressed after a traffic accident. A lateral abdominal film showed a large fluid-dense mass in the retroperitoneal space displacing the intestines ventrally (**A**). Another important radiographic finding was the non-visualization of both kidneys. Because of these findings, excretrory urography was performed. During the nephrogenic phase of the procedure, i.e. the phase immediately following the contrast injection, the "blushed" left kidney proved to be normal while the opacified right kidney showed a severe laceration at the pelvic area (**B**) (arrows). During the excretory phase of the examination, it became clear that the right kidney was producing urine that was spilling into the retroperitoneal space (**C**). The left kidney showed a normal renal pelvis and ureter.*

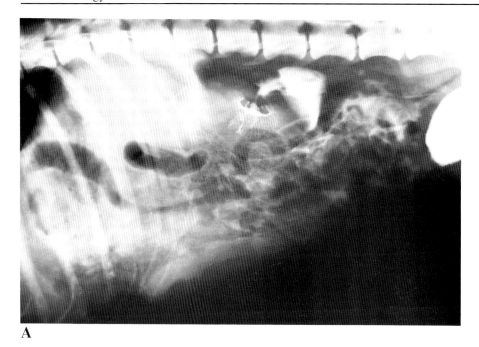

A

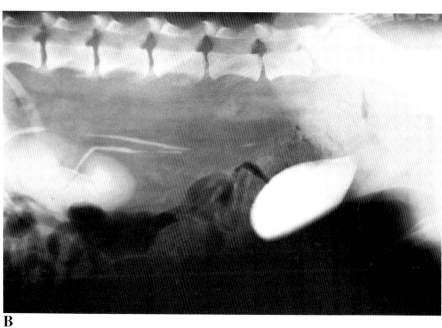

B

Figure 3-14.

Ruptured or normal ureters

*In an adult Toy Poodle, excretory urography proved the presence of a ruptured left ureter with leakage of urine from the retroperitoneal space into the peritoneal cavity (**A**). Bladder opacification is due to normal function and transport of the right kidney and ureter. In a 2-year-old German Shepherd Dog excretory urography proved normal morphology and function of the urologic system (**B**). The large retroperitoneal fluid collection was due to a retroperitoneal hematoma.*

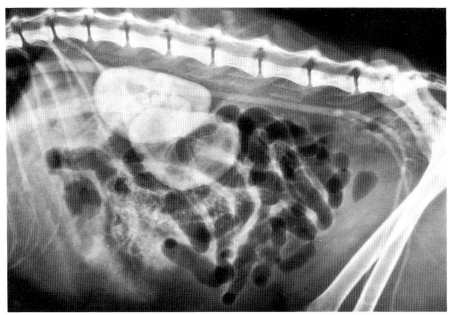

A

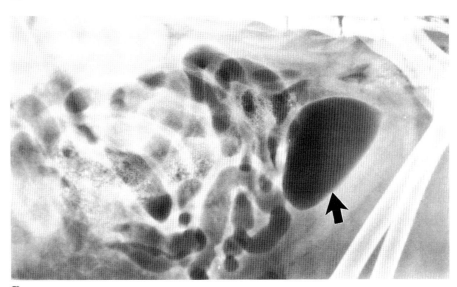

B

Figure 3-15.
Iatrogenic ligation of ureters.
*After spaying, a 1-year-old domestic short-haired cat became increasingly depressed
and uremic. Excretory urography showed normal opacification (blush) of the abdominal vessels and both kidneys immediately following injection (**A**). However, during the
following hours, no excretion of urine containing the injected contrast agent was noticed (**B**). For localization of the bladder, a pneumocystogram was performed (arrow). At the same time, there seemed to be a slight increase in opacity of the abdominal
viscera. Surgery proved that both ureters were ligated obstructing passage of excreted
urine. The generalized increased abdominal opacity was due to the prolonged circula-
tion of the iodinized salts of the contrast medium and the slow excretion by secondary
pathways such as liver and intestines.*

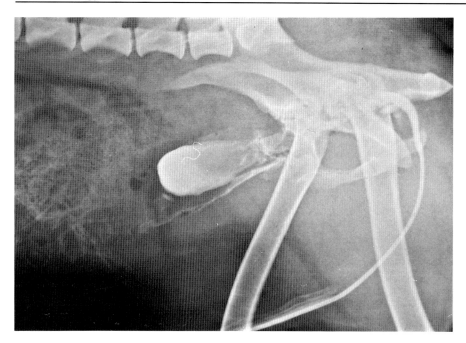

Figure 3-16.
Urinary bladder neck perforation due to pelvic fractures.
A positive-contrast retrograde urethro-cystogram proved the presence of a urinary bladderneck tear in a 3-year-old German Pointer that presented clinical signs of abdominal distension and pain following a traffic accident. One of the pelvic fracture segments had perforated the bladderneck.

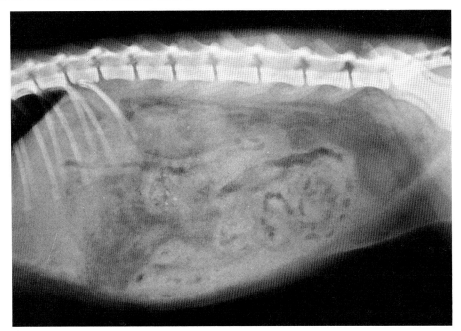

A

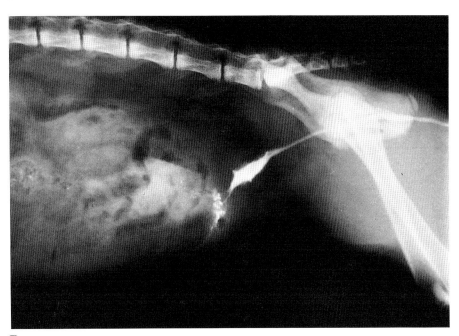

B

Figure 3-17.
Hydroperitoneum due to urinary bladder rupture.
*Following a fall from the third floor of an apartment house, this adult domestic short-
haired cat became depressed and was presented after 3 days with minor abdominal
distension. The lateral radiograph indicates the presence of free peritoneal fluid (**A**).
A positive-contrast cystogram revealed the origin of the hydroperitoneum that was a
rupture of the urinary bladder (**B**).*

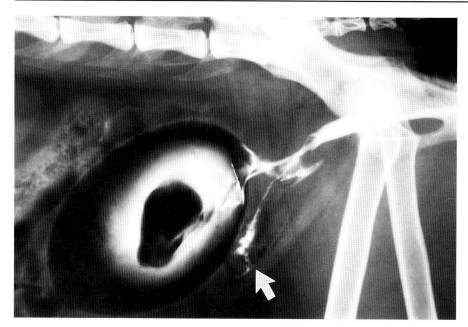

Figure 3-18.
Iatrogenic urethral perforation.
Iatrogenic perforation of the urethra in this 12-year-old domestic short-haired cat during positive-contrast retrograde cystography resulted in retroperitoneal leakage of contrast medium (arrow).

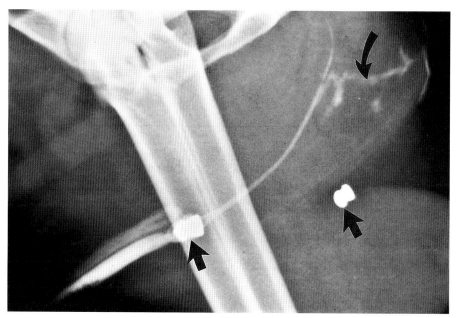

Figure 3-19.
Traumatic urethral perforation.
A 3-year-old cross-breed dog was brought in with a gunshot wound in the perineal region. Fluid thought to be urine was leaking from the wound. A non-contrast radiograph of the area showed 2 separate metallic bullets in the perineal soft tissues (straight arrows). One of these bullets seemed to be lodged at the caudal orifice of the os priapi. A positive-contrast retrograde urethrogram illustrates the intro-urethral position of the bullet and the perforation channel in the perineum (curved arrow) where the bullet had passed through the skin and soft tissues.

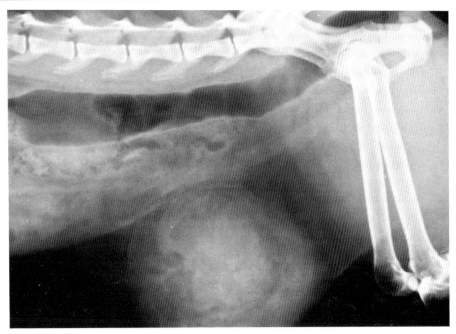

A

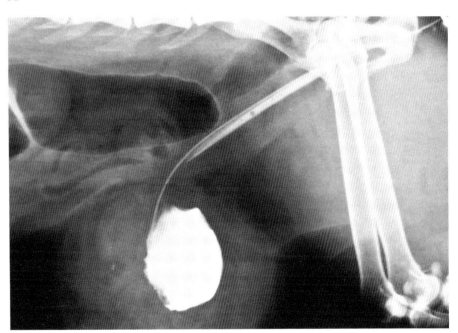

B

Figure 3-20.
Ventral hernia with displaced urinary bladder.
*Dysuria was the main clinical problem of this 12-year-old domestic short-haired cat that had a post-traumatic soft tissue swelling under the ventral body wall. On the lateral abdominal radiograph, the normal intra-abdominal silhouette of the urinary bladder and small intestines was missing (**A**). Catheterization of the urethra and administration of iodine-containing contrast medium revealed the location of the urinary bladder within the ventral hernia (**B**).*

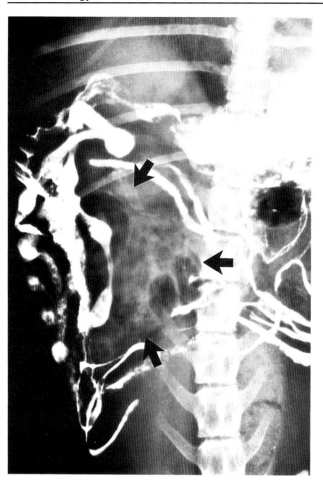

Figure 3-21.
Traumatic pancreatitis.

An adult Schnauzer collapsed several days following blunt abdominal trauma. Clinical signs included a rigid, very painful abdomen. Non-contrast abdominal radiographs revealed a localized, ill-defined increased density within the right epigastric region. A barium study showed an irregular outline of the small bowel loops that seemed to be displaced laterally around an area of increased density (arrows). Traumatic pancreatitis was diagnosed.

IV. RADIOLOGY OF MUSCULOSKELETAL TRAUMA

1. Introduction

Trauma may result in injury to the musculoskeletal system and often causes injury to other organs in the body as well. Following stabilization of the patient, radiographs can be made of the suspected bony lesion. Few fractures, luxations, or other bony lesions are life-threatening, and it must be remembered that attention to the animal must first be directed toward resolving problems associated with blood loss, a compromised airway, or post-traumatic shock. Fractured bones can be immobilized by use of a Robert-Jones bandage or other splinting devices and radiographic studies delayed. Only after the animal is stabilized clinically, is it appropriate to direct one's attention toward the location and character of a bone or joint injury. An exception to this rule may be found in animals with spinal injury in whom a survey radiographic study, often limited to a lateral view, may be necessary to reach answers relative to the necessity of immediate spinal cord decompression or vertebral fracture stabilization. Radiographs made immediately of an animal with head injury may be helpful in the determination of prognosis.

When discussing trauma, the musculoskeletal system is most conveniently divided into the axial and appendicular skeleton. This is helpful because of great variation in radiographic appearance of similar lesions in each division, differences in character of the bony structures between the two divisions, and differences in radiographic techniques used. Injury to diarthrodial joints in the limbs is considered separately because of the difference in radiographic changes and because of the difference in clinical significance of injury to the joints. Even though radiographic evaluation of the soft tissues is limited, some comments are included that may provide additional information in trauma cases. The information presented in this section focuses on the dog as much as the cat, and examples of both species are provided. One major difference between the species is that in the cat

long bones undergo more extensive comminution following trauma.

Radiography of the long bones is easier to perform than studies of the bones of the axial skeleton. Two orthogonal views should be obtained of every animal in an effort to generate a three dimensional picture of the injured tissues. This is essential for the development of a plan that will result in adequate reduction and stability of the fracture/luxation.

Radiographically evident bony changes often occur following trauma at the location of attachment of soft tissues such as the joint capsule, ligaments, and tendons (Figs 4-1, 4-2). The resulting bony spurs are called enthesophytes and appear as a focal lesion rather than the more wide-spread pattern of new bone associated with periosteal elevation (Fig. 4-3). Periosteal elevation occurs in association with or without bone fracture and is identified more commonly in the immature dog or cat because of loose periosteal attachment. Enthesophyte formation is noted in older animals.

2. Axial Skeletal Trauma

Emergency management of trauma to the axial skeleton is a challenge, and morbidity and mortality of these animals remain high. It is important for the clinician to properly advise an owner regarding the method of handling the injured animal during the time of transportation to the clinic. The animal should be placed on a stretcher and secured in a fixed position if either head or spinal cord injury is suspected. Hopefully, radiographs can be made with the animal on this stretcher, avoiding additional patient movement. Radiography is by far the most useful diagnostic aid in determining the nature and exact location of traumatic injuries of the spinal column. However, it is important that the location of the radiographic signs correlates with the expected location as determined by the neurologic examination. If this correlation is not found, additional radiographs or an additional neurologic examination should be conducted. Because multiple spinal injuries may be present, the radiographic study should include the entire vertebral column even when neurologic signs appear to be rather specific in locating the cause of a transverse myelopathy.

The following rules must be followed to obtain correct positioning of the animal for spinal radiography so that evaluation of quality non-contrast radiographs of the spine can lead to a diagnosis. A separate ventrodorsal and lateral radiograph are made of the cervical, the thoracic, the thoracolumbar, and the lumbar regions of animals weighing over 10 kg. The spine of small dogs and cats may be successfully examined radiographically using fewer radiographic sectional views. Radiolucent patient positioning devices are needed to obtain correct positioning of the animal so that the vertebral column is parallel to the table top and rotation of the animal avoided. In the event of an acutely injured animal, it is prudent to make a survey type of examination consisting of several lateral radiographs of the spine. This permits the detection of an fracture/luxation with marked displacement of the vertebral segments. In the event of a fractured spine, it may be useful to use a horizontal X-ray beam to obtain the orthogonal view and avoid physical positioning the patient for a VD or DV view since that might result in further injury to the spinal cord.

A basic rule in radiography of an acutely injured animal is that some degree of malpositioning is tolerable rather than causing further injury to the animal's spinal cord in an effort to obtain perfect radiographic positioning. Additional radiographic studies can be performed later following further clinical examination.

Radiographic examination of the head is compromised because of the differences in shape and size of the head dependent on breed and species. In an effort to overcome this problem of differences in morphology, the radiographic study may ultimately include closed-mouth lateral, open-mouth lateral, dorsoventral, ventrodorsal, closed-mouth lateral oblique, open-mouth lateral oblique, intraoral ventrodorsal, intraoral dorsoventral, open-mouth ventrodorsal, frontal, basal, and occipital views. For the quality of these views to be acceptable, they have to be made on an anesthetized animal. In the event of an animal with serious head injury, anesthesia is probably not possible and therefore, only lateral and dorsoventral views of the head can be made to serve as a survey study. A more complete radiographic study with additional views can be performed at a later time to detect more subtle injuries.

2.1. Fracture location
The axial skeleton includes the mandible, skull and vertebral column. Often injuries to the ribs, sternum, and pelvis are also visualized on skull and vertebral radiographs. The appearance of fractures varies greatly due to anatomical variations and the nature of the injury. Fortunately, it is relatively convenient to obtain radiographic views that permit evaluation of the opposite part for comparison. This is especially true of the ventrodorsal or dorsoventral views. If a suspect lesion is identified on an oblique view, examination of the opposite oblique view makes diagnosis easier by showing that the radiographic change is not present on that view. Still, the presence of fractures of the skull is difficult to ascertain because of the absence of a clearly-visible cortical break that is such a prominent and expected radiographic sign with fractures of long tubular bones. It is possible for trauma to cause injury to more than one part of the axial skeleton. In animals in which this may have occurred, it is important to conduct a complete survey study (Fig. 4-4).

Skull fractures
Because of the character of the skull, trauma causes unique types of fractures. Usually, many small, displaced, bony fragments are noted with the displacement in accordance with the type of injury. If the injury is from a blunt insult, the bony fragments are depressed and are frequently difficult to visualize (Fig. 4-5). Bite wounds due to injury sustained in a big dog-little dog interaction, often cause outward displacement of bony fragments as they are avulsed from their normal location. Because of the heavy bony tissue in the calvarium of many of the larger, heavier breeds, fractures of these bones are relatively uncommon. This is probably also due to the fact that if the injury was severe enough to cause fractures of these bones, it probably caused the immediate death of the animal (Fig. 4-5). It is also possible that trauma to the calvarium causes permanent or transitory neurologic signs without fracturing the bony structures, and the radiographic examination is negative for fractures.

A common site of trauma to the head of larger dogs is within the frontal region because of the prominence of these bones in many breeds. Marked displacement of bony fragments of the frontal bone may be noted and yet the animal only presents with a "headache". The fragments are usually comminuted and depressed. These fractures should be considered open fractures since they open into the air-filled frontal sinuses that usually contain bacteria in large numbers (Fig. 4-5). Another common site of fractures of the head that can be detected radiographically are those within the nasal region. These fractures are evident as lucent lines within the maxilla and premaxilla, but may be difficult to identify because of the associated hemorrhage within the nasal passages that tends to obscure the radiolucent fracture lines (Fig. 4-6).

Fractures of the zygomatic processes are common because of their lateral prominence on the head. Fractures of these bones are relatively easy to identify on the ventrodorsal or dorsoventral view (Fig. 4-7). Fractures of the base of the skull and temporomandibular joints are difficult to assess.

Mandibular fractures

Fractures within the mandible most commonly involve the body and are readily identified radiographically because they resemble, more closely, the fractures of a long bone with disruption of the heavy cortical shadow (Fig. 4-8). Fractures of the ramus of the mandible are much more difficult to identify because of the hindering effect of superimposed bony structures (Fig. 4-9). Symphyseal fractures of the mandible may be more easily detected by physical examination than by radiographic studies. This is especially so when the radiographic examination is performed immediately following the injury, when the animal is often in shock and breathing is compromised by hemorrhage in the nasal passages or in the mouth. If possible, an open-mouth radiograph or intraoral placement of a non-screen film permits more complete evaluation of a symphyseal fracture (Fig. 4-10).

Dental fractures

With any traumatic injury to the head, it is important to assess the teeth and periodontal tissues radiographically for possible fractures (Figs. 4-6 , 4-9, 4-10, 4-11). These radiographic studies are usually made by oblique views, with the animal's mouth opened. Non-screen type dental films can be placed in the mouth and an intra-oral radiographic technique used, thereby improving the quality of the study. However, it may be difficult to insure correct placement of the film. Even following detection of the fracture, it may not be possible to easily ascertain the clinical significance of the dental or periodontal injury (Fig. 4-12).

Spinal fractures and/or luxations

Fractures, luxations, or fracture/luxation of the vertebral column are characterized differently from injury to the head. The radiographic signs of vertebral trauma are summarized (Table 4-1). Malalignment of the vertebral segments is perhaps the most prominent radiographic change noted in traumatized animals. Scoliosis, kyphosis, or lordosis, often with an abrupt "stair-step" form of malalignment may be the result. It is presented as: (1) ventrodorsally or laterally malpositioned vertebral segments, (2) rotationally malpositioned vertebral segments, or (3) malalignment of the floor and roof of the spinal canal. Segmental malalignment may also be detected on the ventrodorsal or dorsoventral views by noting the relative position of the spinal processes. In the normal animal, the spinal processes are positioned in a straight and continuous line and detection of a sudden deviation suggests a traumatically induced malalignment, with or without dynamic instability. Examination of the malaligned vertebral segments may lead to the subtle detection of subluxation of the articular processes that form the vertebral joints

dorsally (Figs. 4-16, 4-17). Associated fractures of the lamina may be present. These traumatic changes in size and shape of the vertebral arch are much less common and more difficult to identify than changes involving the vertebral body (Fig. 4-17).

Table 4-1:
Radiographic signs of vertebral trauma
1. scloliosis, kyphosis, or lordosis (Fig. 4-15)
2. rotational deformity indicated by malpositioned spinal processes (Figs. 4-14, 4-15, 4-17)
3. malalignment between vertebral segments (Figs. 4-13, 4-14, 4-15, 4-16)
4. interruption of the line indicating the floor or roof of the spinal canal (Figs. 4-13, 4-14, 4-15, 4-16)
5. disc space collapse (without degenerative changes) (Figs. 4-13, 4-16)
6. shortened vertebral segments
7. metallic bullet fragments
8. folding cortices of vertebral bodies
9. vertebral endplates not parallel (Fig. 4-13)
10. interrupted vertebral endplates (Fig. 4-14)
11. intrapelvic hemorrhage

Shortened vertebral segments are the result of impaction of the bone due to trauma. Compression fractures cause a change in the size and shape of the vertebral body as well as an increase in density due to bony tissue collapse (Figs. 4-17, 4-18). Trauma may cause only a compression fracture of a vertebral body without any malalignment or rotational deformity, and the resulting change in size, shape, and density of the vertebral body must be differentiated from changes due to tumor, infection, or congenital or developmental lesions (Figs. 4-19, 4-20).

Trauma to the spine may cause disc herniation without obvious fracture or with only minimal bony fragmentation. Collapse of the intervertebral disc space commonly occurs due to disc injury with or without associated vertebral fractures that originate from the "corners" of the vertebral bodies (Fig. 4-13). Examination of the vertebral endplates helps in separating acute traumatic disc space collapse from that seen in association with chronic disc disease. Disc space collapse associated with chronic degeneration of the intervertebral disc leads secondarily to development of sclerosis of the vertebral endplates and production of reactive vertebral osteophytes (Figs. 4-13, 4-19). Disc space collapse associated with acute injury does not show the classical degenerative changes (Fig. 4-13). It also occurs in association with developmental disease (Fig. 4-19).

In some animals that present with signs of cord compression, collapse of the disc space or malalignment is not obvious. Because of the absence of radiographic changes seen on the non-contrast radiographs, myelography is necessary to identify the protruded disc tissue that is acting as an extradural mass causing a transverse myelopathy (Figs. 4-21, 4-22). The myelogram may also detect dural tearing through the detection of contrast medium leakage.

Additional radiographic patterns associated with trauma to the spine include the presence of metallic fragments associated with a gunshot injury (Figs. 4-23, 4-24). The character of the metallic shadows is dependent on the nature of the bullet and its velocity at the moment of impact. Another radiographic pattern is associated with pathologic fractures in which "folding" cortices secondary to osteopenic bone are noted (Fig. 4-25).

Traumatic injury to the vertebral column rarely produces a perivertebral soft tissue shadow radiographically that is associated with the resulting hemorrhage and edema. An exception to this rule occurs with a fracture of the sacrum or caudal vertebrae in which the blood pools in the retroperitoneal space within the pelvic canal, dorsal to the rectum (Fig. 4-26).

A very unique spinal injury is that lesion where fractured lamina are separated from the vertebral body. This is important to notice radiographically because this type of fracture may cause "self decompression" of the spinal canal by providing space for the spinal cord without cord compression. Understanding of this radiographic sign allows for a more thorough examination of the vertebral column (Fig. 4-27).

Dynamic or stress radiography of the axial skeleton involves the use of flexion and extension views for further evaluation of a region of questionable vertebral instability, and is often helpful in demonstrating the degree of the instability, degree of cord compression, and the presence of possible associated fractures. Stress views are most often used in examination of the occipito-atlanto-axial region (Fig. 4-28), the cervical region, and the lumbosacral junction (Fig. 4-29). This type of special radiographic positioning includes hyperflexed and hyperextended positioning or exaggerated lateral positioning to show malalignment and instability of vertebral segments. It must be performed with extreme care to avoid further compressive injury to the spinal cord. It is most important to remember that the patient is probably anesthetized or, if not anesthetized, unable to resist manipulation of the spine at the time of the radiographic examination, and any unusual or excessive efforts at flexion or extension may exacerbate the neurological injury. However, there is a balance to be achieved between the necessity to learn the information which the

stress radiographs can provide and the possible exacerbation of the injury.

Lumbosacral fractures and/or luxations

Injury to the nerve roots within the lumbosacral region is less common than expected because of the tapering of the cauda equina. Still, cauda equina syndrome is regularly identified in both dogs and cats. The nerve roots have a relatively small cross-sectional measurement that enables them to lie within a bony canal that permits rather marked displacement of the vertebral segments and still does not result in serious compressive injury to the cord or spinal nerves. Injury may be exacerbated in certain animals because of a spinal canal that is congenitally smaller than normal providing a smaller cross section in which the cauda equina must fit. This vertebral canal stenosis may be due to a congenital anomaly, while in older animals the injury is often superimposed over a herniated intervertebral disc that has undergone degenerative changes associated with chronic disc disease. It may be difficult to determine whether the malalignment between the last lumbar segment and the sacrum is traumatically induced or is due to disc degeneration (Fig. 4-30). Fractures of the body of the seventh lumbar vertebra can also cause injury to the nerve roots and are relatively easy to identify radiographically, but fractures of the sacrum that can cause similar clinical signs are more difficult to visualize. Often, the latter are more laterally directed and are best seen on ventrodorsal views as they extend into the wings of the sacrum (Fig. 4-31).

Rib fractures

Fractures of the ribs received a detailed treatment in the section on thoracic trauma since they play an important role in injury to the chest wall, and are often a cause of pneumothorax as well as hemorrhage into the pleural space and lungs. They occur commonly as the result of traffic accidents, falls, crushing bite wounds, or sharp blows to the chest wall. Detection of the fractures depends on noticing the displacement of the fracture fragments with identification of a radiolucent space between the fragment ends as well as a definite alteration in the normal contour of the affected rib. If the ends of the bony fragments remain closely positioned, they may overlap and produce a more radiodense shadow (Figs. 4-32, 4-33). In that situation, alteration in the contour of the rib is less obvious. Depending on the nature of the trauma, the fractures may be similarly placed on both sides of the chest wall, suggesting penetrating bite wounds. With more blunt trauma, the fractures involve adjacent ribs in only one chest wall. If there are two fractures each in adjacent ribs, a segment of thoracic wall is separated and moves in a paradoxical direction with respiration. This is called a "flail" chest and can seriously compromise the ability of the animal to breathe. However, in most traumatized animals, the soft tissue injury to the chest wall and lung is more important than the rib fractures. In older animals, fractures of the calcified costal arches are difficult to diagnose because of the rather bizarre radiographic pattern of degenerative calcified tissue at the costochondral junction that extends into the costal arches as well.

Sternal fractures and/or luxations

Sternal fracture/dislocations are a unique injury (Fig. 4-34). The sternal segments are not weight-bearing, and clinical signs associated with their injury are often minimal. Because of location, injury to the sternal segments indicates possible associated injury to the chest wall, and the detection of injury to the sternum should direct careful attention to the remainder of the thorax as it is examined for more clinically significant lesions. Because of the adjacent internal thoracic vessels, it could be assumed that sternal fractures with displacement might be associated with severe pleural hemorrhage. However, this is rarely noted. Congenital sternal anomalies are common in the region of the xiphoid cartilage, and radiographic interpretation of abnormalities in this region should be done carefully (Fig. 4-35).

Pelvic fractures

Fractures of the pelvis are unique because of its basic anatomical structure. The "ring" or "box" concept aids in understanding the pattern of fractures or luxations. Because of this morphology, trauma to the pelvis usually results in three separate but related lesions involving the ilium, pubis, and ischium on the same side, or involving both sides. Another pattern that is frequently seen is the combination of two bony fractures plus a sacroiliac or pubic symphyseal separation (Fig. 4-36). A less common pattern of injury occurs when the two halves of the pelvis separate, with fracture of one sacroiliac joint and separation of the pubic symphysis (Fig. 4-26). It is also possible to have an acetabular fracture plus a sacroiliac separation that divides the pelvis into two halves (Fig. 4-37). Both sacroiliac joints can be luxated and separate the intact bony pelvis from the sacrum. This is often seen in cats and it is important in these animals with sacroiliac injury to investigate whether the sacrum is fractured. Involvement of the wings of the sacrum is difficult to determine radiographically but is clinically important because of potential physical instability as well as the possibility of injury to the cauda equina (Fig. 4-31). Fractures entering the acetabulum destroy the contour of that joint, and even with fragment healing, secondary joint disease will develop because of the persistent disruption of the contour of the joint surface (Figs. 4-38, 4-39, 4-40). The radiographic signs of pelvic trauma are listed in Table 4-2.

Additional injury to the neighboring bony structures is possible with pelvic fractures. Avulsion of the apophyseal centers of the ilial and the ischial crest can be found in the younger animals in whom skeletal maturation has not oc-

Table 4-2:
Radiographic signs of pelvic trauma
1. pattern of fractures involving the ileum, pubis, and ischium on the same side or involving both sides
2. bilateral or unilateral sacro-iliac separation (Figs. 4-36, 4-37)
3. acetabular fractures (Figs. 4-37, 4-38, 4-39)
4. avulsion of ilial and ischial crest apophyseal centers
5. sacral fractures
6. sacro-coccygeal luxation
7. coccygeal luxation
8. intrapelvic hemorrhage
9. cranial displacement of the hemipelvis (Fig. 4-36)
10. narrowed pelvic canal
11. additional fractures (Figs. 4-41, 4-42)

curred. This is usually without accompanying clinical signs. Because of the closeness of the proximal femur, any patient with an injury to the pelvis needs to have the femoral head, femoral neck, and greater trochanter closely evaluated by physical examination and by radiographic examination (Fig. 4-41). Traumatic separation of the sacral segments or fracture/luxation of the caudal segments often occurs simultaneously with trauma of the pelvis, and needs to be detected since this injury may be associated with paresis or paralysis of the tail (Fig. 4-42).

2.2. Osteomyelitis

Infection in the bones of the head is usually associated with puncture-type injuries (Fig. 4-43). Even if the fractures extend into the nasal cavity or paranasal sinuses, making them open fractures, the frequency of osteomyelitis is low. Fractures into the oral cavity more often become infected. This causes special problems for the treatment of the fractures that extend into the periodontal space.

Bone infection in the spine may occur secondary to trauma. However, it is difficult to predict what kind of injury will induce secondary bone infection. It can be the direct effect of a penetrating wound, but also the result of hematogenous osteomyelitis. The latter may have a post-traumatic or post-surgical pathogenesis. Osteomyelitis is difficult to detect in the cancellous bone tissue of the vertebral body because there is little sclerotic response around the destructive lesion that would be helpful for radiographic diagnosis. The early radiographic changes of osteomyelitis in the presence of a fracture are even more difficult to ascertain because of the expected presence of overlying callus formation associated with the fracture. Usually, the diagnosis of osteomyelitis is first made on the basis of the clinical signs. When the infection has progressed to the point of causing destruction of the vertebral endplates or has caused marked reactive bony production, the radiographic changes are more prominent but may still be confused with those associated with a healing fracture (Fig. 4-44). A similar diagnostic problem exists in the event of a spinal luxation that is secondarily infected. The bony response to the original injury appears as new periosteal bone formation plus soft tissue calcification. These changes are superimposed over the new bone production associated with the infection, making diagnosis difficult.

3. Appendicular Skeletal Trauma

Diagnostic radiology is conveniently used in clinical practice for the diagnosis of fractures of long bones and for the determination of the prognosis of fracture healing. A fracture within a long bone is best defined as a lesion causing an interruption of the continuity of the bone resulting from stress that is beyond the capacity of the bone to withstand. The radiographic study must include the joints that are proximal and distal to the injury and should include two orthogonal views. Only on a complete radiographic study can the full character of the fracture be determined and the possible involvement of the adjacent joints be evaluated. Both the character of the soft tissue injury as well as the nature of the bony injury should be evaluated on the radiographs. The degree of soft tissue injury partially determines the healing potential of the fracture. With severe soft tissue injury, the new extra-periosteal blood supply that feeds the healing fracture fails to form and delayed fracture healing or a non-union fracture results. Information on the nature of the soft tissue injury can be estimated from the radiograph by noting the amount of swelling and hematoma formation as well as the displacement of the fracture fragments. In addition, detection of the presence of interposed soft tissues that separate the bony fragments are an indication of a potential delay to the fracture healing. Marked fragment overriding or severe comminution of the fragments are other indications of extensive soft tissue injury and potential delay in healing. The radiograph, at best, offers only a clue to the extent of soft tissue injury, but should be judged as closely as possible, since it is an valuable addition to the physical examination.

3.1. Fracture classification
Fracture classification is based on the completeness of the fracture line, the number of fracture lines, and the location of the fragments (Table 4-3). Critical evaluation of the character of a fracture and classification permits assessment of the opportunities for "normal" fracture healing as well as determination of the fixation method to be utilized. In addition, the underlying character of the bone involved needs to be examined carefully to avoid overlooking a pathological fracture. Obviously, the determination of

fracture type is much easier within a long bone than it is in a bone in the axial skeleton where the shape and size of the bones vary widely.

Physeal fractures
Physeal fractures are unique injuries frequently seen in the skeletally immature animal. Because the growth region of the long bone is damaged there is the potential for alteration to the normal growth pattern of the bone. The classification of physeal fractures is described on the basis of involvement of the physis, metaphysis, and epiphysis.

In the simplest form (**Type-I**), a physeal fracture consists of injury to the replicating cartilaginous cells in the physis with the bony fragments returning to their normal anatomical positioning after the injury or remaining with various degrees of fragment malposition (Figs. 4-45, 4-46). This type of injury is common in bones that have a plate-like physis and separation can take place without injury to the metaphysis. It occurs commonly within the distal radius, proximal femur, and the proximal humerus.

More severe injury to the bone (physis) results in greater displacement of the fragments or the presence of fracture lines within the epiphysis, the metaphysis, or both. The fracture line may escape from the physis, run into the metaphysis, and separate a small triangular shaped bony fragment from the metaphysis (**Type-II**) (Fig. 4-47). This injury is common in physes that have an undulating surface, often with four pyramidal-shaped protrusions that fit into four depressions establishing strength to the growth region. This fracture occurs commonly in the distal femur, distal humerus, and the proximal tibia.

Another physeal fracture involves the physis in part but turns and passes through the epiphysis. This fracture (**Type-III**) is articular in addition to involving the growth plate (Fig. 4-48). It is uncommon, but is seen in the distal humerus, the distal radius, and the proximal tibia.

The physeal injury may be more longitudinally directed, with the fracture line passing through the epiphysis, across the physis, and into the metaphysis exiting a short distance from the physeal plate (Figs. 4-49, 4-50). This fracture (**Type-IV**) is commonly seen in the distal humerus.

An additional physeal injury occurs when the injury causes a crushing injury to the growth plate and periphyseal bony bridging occurs that prevents normal growth in length of the bone (**Type-V**). This is typical of injuries to the distal ulna.

An important consequence of bony injury involving the physes results from the possible interruption of normal

Table 4-3: **Fracture classification based on radiographic examination**

A. *Number of fracture lines*

1. A **simple fracture** is characterized by a lack of comminution, the presence of only one fracture line, and may be complete or incomplete:

   a. complete – fracture line extends through the bone involving the entire cortex (both cortical shadows are interrupted as seen on a single radiographic view)

   b. incomplete – fracture line does not involve the entire cross-section of the bone and a portion of the cortex remains intact (only one cortical shadow is interrupted as seen on one of the orthogonal radiographic views)

      1) *greenstick fracture* is common in immature bones

      2) *buckling fracture* occurs in bones weakened by pathologic process

      3) *impacted fracture* occurs more commonly in cancellous bone of the metaphyses as trabeculae are driven into each other and a distinct radiolucent fracture line is not identified

      4) *penetration fracture* is due to penetration of a foreign body (such as a bullet) and causes an incomplete fracture due to injury to only one cortex

      5) *stress fracture* occurs in a bone experiencing repeated stress cycling and has a fracture line extending only partially through the bone involving only one cortex

2. A **multiple fracture** is a pattern of complete simple fractures characterized by more than one major fracture line within a bone.

3. A **comminuted fracture** is a complete fracture characterized by additional fracture lines creating multiple small bone fragments, in addition to those created by the major fracture line(s). If the fragments are large, the fracture may be referred to as a multiple fracture.

B. *Direction or character of fracture lines*
These may vary widely and are described as:

1. oblique
2. spiral
3. transverse
4. avulsion
5. saucer
6. fissure or longitudinal
7. stress

C. *Location of fracture line(s)*
These are described as:

1. diaphyseal
2. metaphyseal
3. epiphyseal/metaphyseal
4. epiphyseal (or articular), involving subchondral bone
5. physeal (skeletally immature patient)

D. *Relationship of fracture fragments*
Described in terms of:

1. degree of end-to-end apposition of fragments
2. alignment of the fragments relative to adjacent joints and weight-bearing surfaces
3. degree of angulation between the fragments
4. degree of rotation between the fragments
5. presence and extent of overall bone shortening

E. *Associated joint injury*
These may be due to :

1. fracture line entering the joint space
2. combination of fracture/luxation
3. avulsion or intra-articular corner fragments

F. *Soft tissue injury*
This is characterized by:

1. closed fracture with no break in adjacent skin
2. open fracture with a break in adjacent skin characterized by
   a. free air within soft tissues
   b. bone fragments protruding through a break in skin
   c. radiopaque debris within soft tissues due to surface contaminants or a foreign body e.g. bullet
3. interposition of soft tissues between bony fragments
4. swelling due to edema/hematoma
5. suspect injury to nutrient artery
6. suspect injury to nerve

---

bone growth. This interruption may cause premature closure within a growth plate, with resulting cessation of growth or interruption of growth which may be temporary, with normal or near-normal growth recurring later. These interruptions in normal growth patterns may involve all or a part of the affected physis. These injuries to the growth potential of the bone may result in shortening of the affected bone with or without angular deformity, depending on the part of the physis affected and the duration and extent of the effect.

When this type of growth abnormality occurs within a single bone, lameness or alteration in gait is seldom noticed. However, when it occurs in one of a pair of bones, the effect is serious, requiring surgical intervention. Because of the near-equal size of the radius and ulna, injury to the growth areas in the distal forelimb results in a remarkable clinical problem whereby growth in one of the bones is inhibited and growth in the other bone continues at a near-normal rate. Following injury to a growth plate in the radius and/or ulna, abnormal (decreased) bone growth in one of the paired bones will probably occur resulting in unequal growth of the two bones, with consequent bowing of the unaffected bone which continues to grow in a normal manner. This comparatively longer bone causes failure of development of normal articular surfaces and marked injury to the developing antebrachiocarpal or elbow joint. The other possible result of unequal growth between the radius and ulna is that the unaffected bone continues to grow, remaining straight, and causes a subluxation of the elbow or antebrachiocarpal joint with a resulting severe deforming arthrosis. Most of the time, this type of injury results in a shortened ulna with injury to the radio-carpal joint (Figs. 4-51, 4-52, 4-53). Injury to the elbow joint is less common (Fig. 4-54). It is also possible for both radio-carpal and elbow joints to be affected secondarily (Fig. 4-55). Occasionally, development of these lesions is complicated by the presence of synostosis between the pair of growing bones.

Shortening of the radius as compared with the ulna is less common (Fig. 4-56).

Repeated clinical and radiographic examinations are necessary for accurate evaluation of potential growth abnormalities because of the rapid rate of growth of long bones in immature dogs and cats. The time between the original injury causing the physeal growth disturbance and the detection of bowing of the limb is short, often between 2 and 4 weeks. Thus, unless the owner is advised of this potential growth problem, injury to the adjacent joints may occur prior to the moment that the owner asks for medical assistance. Correct diagnosis of the original traumatic injury or detection of early secondary changes is obviously important in determining prognosis for an animal that may only be beginning to show abnormalities and is also important in determining the time and need for orthopedic surgery in the more severely affected patient.

Apophyseal avulsion fractures
Avulsion of apophyseal growth centers is a rather frequently occurring injury following trauma, with the bony fragment displaced proximally away from the parent bone. This type of injury is commonly associated with the suprascapular tuberosity, the greater trochanter of the femur, the tibial crest, and the ossification center for the olecranon process (Figs. 4-57, 4-58). The apophysis usually does not fragment and can be re-attached to the parent bone by means of a small metallic screw or K-E wire and stabilized by use of a tension-band device during healing. Usually, the bony portion of the apophyseal growth center

does not fracture since the cartilage plate separating the apophysis from the parent bone is the area of greatest weakness and, consequently, the fracture lines are limited to that region. There is no predisposing reason for the separation and therefore the injuries are usually unilateral.

Because apophyseal growth lines do not contribute prominently to the length of the bone, perfect repositioning of the avulsed fragment that leads to renewed physeal growth is not required. Separation of the tibial crest is unique since avulsion alters the length of the patellar ligament and, in that way, may influence the matching of the femoropatellar joint. Because of the available soft tissue blood supply, most apophyseal center avulsion fractures heal easily following repositioning. Additional traction type injuries involve the growth centers of the accessory carpal bone, the calcaneus, the lesser trochanter of the femur, the supraglenoid tubercle of the scapula, the greater trochanter of the humerus, and the medial epicondyle of the humerus.

Osteochondrosis of the tibial tuberosity in man is referred to by the eponym "Osgood Schlatter's" disease. However, in dogs and cats, avulsion of the tibial tuberosity is a traumatic injury to normally developing bone and is not an osteochondrosis type injury.

The possibility of concomitant joint injury is remote because this type of injury is away from the articular surface and extracapsular in location. For that reason, every effort should be made to keep the surgical repositioning of the apophyses extracapsular as well. In cases of tibial crest avulsion, injury to the femoropatellar joint is possible because of the displacement of the patella proximally. Repositioning of the avulsed fragment should be made with the purpose of reducing the patellar luxation so that it again articulates with the trochlear groove of the distal femur.

Gunshot injuries
Depending on the culture of a society, gunshot injuries may be more or less common. The missiles range from a small "B-B" or air-gun pellet to numerous lead pellets from a shot-cartridge or to a single high-velocity missile. Most of the lower velocity projectiles only cause soft tissue injury, although an air-gun pellet fired at close range can cause a fracture of a long bone in a cat (Fig. 4-59).

The high-velocity missile from a hunting weapon causes extreme tissue injury, and resulting fractures are usually highly comminuted with associated severe soft tissue injury. The wounding effect of such missiles varies, depending upon mass, shape, velocity, deformation, and whether the missile tumbles or breaks. Velocity is the most important factor. When a bullet strikes a solid object, all or part of its kinetic energy is transmitted to the tissue. Particles of bone accelerate forward and act as secondary missiles. One of the primary features of all missile wounds is cavitation. Within milliseconds after a high-velocity missile impacts and perforates, a pulsating undulating temporary cavity is formed. The surrounding tissue is subsequently explosively pushed and compressed laterally to enclose the temporarily formed cavity. The maximum diameter of this temporary cavity may be approximately 30 times the size of the original missile tract. Therefore, tissues at a distance from the original wound may be damaged and adjacent bones may be fractured without ever having been struck directly by the missile. Lower-velocity missiles create a direct pathway of destruction, with little injury to surrounding tissues.

If the missile is an expanding type, it mushrooms on impact with tissue, so there are multiple metallic fragments (Figs. 4-6-, 4-61) and the tract of the bullet can be identified by the deposition of varying sized lead fragments as the bullet passes through the soft tissues, especially if the bullet is soft. The bullet tract through the patient's body should be determined either radiographically or clinically, so that other organs that are suspected to be injured can be identified and evaluated in addition to the fractures seen radiographically.

The pattern of healing of fractures due to gunshot wounds is dependent on the in-growth of a new blood supply from the damaged surrounding soft tissues, and the bony and metallic fragments, even when left in position, do not seem to adversely affect healing to a degree that might be expected.

Low-velocity missiles such as hail pellets are seen commonly on radiographs, with most of the shot pellets remaining within the subcutis. However, if the injury follows a close-range shotgun blast, massive destruction of soft tissues and bones may occur (Fig. 4-62).

Occasionally an animal is injured when struck by an arrow or dart. Injury by this type of low-velocity missile is uncommon and is more easily detected because of the external protrusion of a part of the missile.

3.2. Fracture location

Scapula
Fractures of the proximal portion, the spine or blade, of the scapula often result from a car passing over the patient's body and result in linear fracture lines with fragments being bent or folded. Radiographic diagnosis of the fractures is difficult because there are no strong cortical shadows that are interrupted. Because of the flattened character of the bone, most fractures result in superimposition of bony fragments with the appearance of lines of increased density within the bone. The clinical significance of any of these fractures is minimal unless the neck is involved, with or without articular involvement through the glenoid cavity

(Fig. 4-63). Therefore, the glenoid cavity should be carefully examined for intra-articular fracture lines. Radiography of the scapula in the traumatized animal may be limited to lateral projections only, made with the unaffected limb retracted cranially or caudally. The orthogonal view requires pulling the leg cranially as far as is possible and this type of positioning is not always possible.

A specific type of injury is an avulsion of the supraglenoid tuberculum with displacement of the free fragment within the soft tissues cranially. This is most commonly seen in young, immature animals.

Humerus
Most fractures of the humerus involve the midshaft and distal portion of this bone. The midshaft fractures are typically spiral in character, often with comminution or butterfly fragments, while the distal fractures involve the distal condylar region creating "T" or "Y" fractures that are intra-articular (Fig. 4-64). Oblique positioning may assist in determining the exact nature of these fracture lines. In skeletally immature animals, ossification centers for the capitulum and the trochlea may be separate following trauma, forming two fragments that need to be reattached before the reunited epiphysis can be fixed to the metaphysis. Physeal fractures of the proximal and distal humerus are usually both Type-I or Type-II (Fig. 4-50).

Radius
This is one of the more commonly fractured bones in the dog and cat, and fractures of almost any description can occur. The majority of radial fractures also have an associated ulnar fracture (Figs. 4-65, 4-66, 4-67). The majority of fractures occur in the midshaft and distal parts of the bone, and rarely include an articular component. Physeal fractures may occur both proximally and distally, but are not commonly detected at the time of injury (Fig. 4-46).

Ulna
Ulnar fractures are common and frequently occur in conjunction with radial fractures. While distal fractures are common, a separate group of fractures involve the olecranon and the olecranon process in the immature patient (Fig. 4-68). Fractures of the styloid process are often seen in combination with a radial fracture and cause instability of the antebracheocarpal joint.

Carpus and phalanges
The small carpal bones are often crushed and radiography should include four views to completely evaluate the fractures. Stress views may help in separating overlying bones so that fractures and sites of instability can be seen more easily. Because of the absence of prominent cortical shadows, carpal fractures are more difficult to see. The metacarpal and proximal and middle phalanges are tubular and,

fractures are more easily noted (Fig. 4-69). The distal phalanx is difficult to position for radiography and a "paddle"
technique forcing the foot flat against the table top may assist in achieving better positioning. Fractures of the proximal sesamoid bones at the metacarpal-phalangeal joints are
a distinct type of injury to the foot and are important clinically (Fig. 4-70).

Femur
The femur is a frequently fractured bone with a wide variety of fracture types. In the young animal, Type-I physeal
fractures involve the femoral head (Fig. 4-45), but are also
common distally (Fig. 4.47). In the immature animal, the
slipped capital epiphysis usually loses its blood supply and
undergoes necrosis. In the adult animal, it is important to
note whether femoral neck fractures are intra- or
extracapsular since this determines to some degree a possible disruption of vascular supply to the femoral head and
neck and, as a result, the possibility of aseptic necrosis.

Articular fractures are uncommon proximally but do occur
distally, with separation of a femoral condyle (Fig. 4-49).
Midshaft fractures result in marked displacement and over-riding of comminuted or butterfly fragments (Figs. 4-71, 4-72).

Positioning for radiography is difficult because of problems in extending the fractured leg when the animal is in
dorsal recumbency. It is possible to make this view with the
limb in a flexed position, referred to as a "frog-leg" position. It is also possible to obtain a craniocaudal view by
putting the animal in a "sitting" position and pulling the
foot distally. Another technique is to partially diagnose the
character of the fracture on the lateral view and delay making the second orthogonal view until a later time when the
animal is anesthetized for surgery.

Tibia
Fractures of the tibia are common, with many different
types seen. In the immature animal, Type-II physeal fractures of the proximal epiphysis are very common. Midshaft
fractures are often oblique and comminuted or have large
butterfly fragments (Fig. 4-73). Distally, fractures of the
medial malleolus may be associated with tibiotarsal
luxations. Fibular fractures are often found in association
with tibial fractures. Unfortunately, if the fibula is intact, it
does not provide enough splinting to be of great value in
stabilization of the tibial fracture.

Tarsus and phalanges
Diagnosis and problems are similar to those noted in the
distal portion of the forelimb.

3.3.   Other traumatically induced skeletal diseases
Osteomyelitis
Bone infection may be associated with open fractures,
however, it is difficult to predict at the time of the original

injury which fractures may be so affected. The possibility
of hematogenous osteomyelitis at the site of a closed fracture due to extensive soft tissue injury also makes the pre-
diction of possible infection through this route difficult. A
third possibility of infection may result from surgical
trauma to the soft tissues during a prolonged reduction/
stabilization intervention. This form of osteomyelitis may
be due to a break in aseptic technique at the time of surgery,
but more likely is due to the degree of soft tissue injury and
secondary hematogenous osteomyelitis. Bone infection
may also be secondary to a primary soft tissue infection
(Figs. 4-74, 4-75).

The early radiographic changes of osteomyelitis in the
presence of a healing fracture are difficult to ascertain because of the frequently found exuberant callus formation
that "covers" the destructive lesion. Any reactive bone associated with the bone infection can therefore be misdiagnosed because it is assumed to be associated with the fracture healing. For these reasons, the diagnosis of osteomyelitis is most often first made on the basis of the clinical
signs which include heat, soft tissue swelling, and formation of a drainage tract.

If the fracture has been stabilized by metallic devices, the
infectious process often centers around the interface between the bone and the metallic implant. Lytic areas are
noted around pins, screws, or plates. The presence of these
destructive areas that may be somewhat randomly located
is highly suggestive of infection (Fig. 4-76). As a result, it is
possible for the metallic devices to become less securely attached to the bone and to move in position. This is especially noticeable when screws "back-out". A differential
diagnosis for lucency around pins is bone erosion associated with movement of the pins. Lucency due to pin motion
has a uniform pattern and involves the bone tissue around
the entire pin.

Post-traumatic aseptic necrosis
Post-traumatic aseptic necrosis is a characteristic lesion that
is noted at anatomical sites where it is possible for a fragment
of bone to be isolated and deprived of its blood supply at the
time of the injury. By that description, it is another manifes-
tation of bone infarction. Generally it is the result of laceration, thrombosis, embolus, or endarteritis affecting the nutrient blood vessels. This type of lesion occurs most commonly
in the capital epiphysis of the femur as a result of interruption
of the major blood supply which is extracapsular and therefore, highly vulnerable to trauma. With physeal separation
of the femoral head in the skeletally immature animal or with
a high intra-articular femoral neck fracture in the skeletally
mature animal, the potential of blood supply through the
femoral neck is cut off, and the blood supply that courses
over the surface of the femoral neck within the soft tissues is interrupted as well. This leaves the femoral head
and possibly a segment of the proximal femoral neck

with a blood supply limited to that passing through the ligament of the femoral head. This supplies only the bone tissue immediately around this ligamentous attachment. Because of this, intra-articular femoral neck fractures or slipped capital epiphyses are important clinically (Fig. 4-77) and healing may not be satisfactory, even with stable fragment reduction. Occasionally, the fracture site is just distal to the capsular attachment and the blood supply to the capital epiphysis is maintained and a more nearly normal healing occurs (Fig. 4-78). The humeral head is also intracapsular but aseptic necrosis following trauma is not often recognized in this bone. Carpal and tarsal bones probably have solitary blood supplies that, following fracture, could result in an avascular fragment. This type of lesion is common in man, but uncommon in the dog or cat.

Spontaneous aseptic necrosis
A lesion somewhat similar to post-traumatic aseptic necrosis occurs spontaneously, or probably in the event of chronic low-grade trauma, as bilateral aseptic necrosis of the femoral heads in smaller breeds of dogs at 6-9 months of age. Often, the lesions cause unilateral clinical signs, but the disease is frequently present bilaterally on histological examination (Fig. 4-79). This lesion is thought to have an insidious kind of development without acute loss of the entire blood supply to the femoral head at one time. Death of bony tissue occurs in only a part of the femoral head at one time, and active osteoblastic activity occurs at the same time as osteoclastic activity. Thus, the reparative process results in production of a femoral head that is somewhat malformed but contains new viable bone tissue and remains within the acetabulum (Fig. 4-80). As a result of the deformity of the articular contour, secondary deforming arthrosis develops with age.

Post-traumatic osteoporosis
Bone atrophy is often associated with apparently minimal bone injury and is called post-traumatic osteoporosis (Sudek's atrophy in man). While this pattern of bone decalcification is well characterized in man, it is incompletely described in animals. It is assumed to be a vasomotor response initiated by pain impulses. The bones of the feet appear to be the most common site of involvement, with cloudy or patchy osteoporosis progressing to an image of reduced, rarefied trabeculae and cortical thinning, eventually leading to complete disappearance of the bone (Fig. 4-81).

Bone infarction
An uncommon bone disease is bone infarction that results from an obstruction in the circulatory system of bone, with consequent necrosis within the marrow cavity. Infarcts may be solitary but usually present as multiple medullary calcifications appearing as confluent or chainlike densities within the distal ends of the radius and tibia (Fig. 4-82). They are rarely diaphyseal. The exact etiology or clinical significance of this condition in animals is not well described. It is occasionally associated with primary malignant bone tumors, but is of little clinical significance.

Trophic bone defects
Detailed information is lacking about the radiographic appearance and clinical significance of electrical or thermal burns, freezing injuries, or long-term injuries resulting from compression of the foot, such as would occur in a trap or a tight cast. These injuries may be referred to as trophic bone defects, meaning only that they are related to the vascular nutrition of a segment of the bone. The radiographic changes are usually those of bone necrosis with periosteal new bone formation (Fig. 4-83). It is often difficult to determine whether the bone necrosis is the result of the original trauma to the bone or the result of injury to the vascular system or nerve supply of the bone. Fortunately, these types of injuries are uncommon and diagnosis or treatment is not often required.

Radiation injury
Radiation injury to bone causes death of the bone tissue without clear demarcation with the adjacent viable bone. Radiation injury has been reported in animals in association with experimental studies on the toxic effects that would occur from exposure by internal alpha-particle or beta-particle emitters such as radium or strontium (Fig. 4-84). Another type of radiation injury in animals may be associated with the use of orthovoltage radiation therapy in the treatment of malignant disease. Radiographic evaluation of the injury is complicated by pre-therapy surgical debulking, possible recurrence of the tumor, or the presence of secondary osteomyelitis.

3.4. Orthopedic fixation devices
Orthopedic fixation devices are used in the treatment of fractures, soft-tissue injuries, and reconstructive sugery. After fracture reduction, internal, external, or intramedullary fixation devices may be used to provide stability and maintain the alignment of bone fragments during the healing process. Screws are used primarily to provide interfragmental compression or to attach plates, which can then provide compression, prevent displacement, and support the fragments during healing. Pins and wires can be used for fixation of small fragments and small bone fractures, for attachment of external fixation devices, and for intramedullary placement in long bone fractures. The use of these devices only became possible with the discovery of X-rays, availability of anesthetics, and an understanding of surgical asepsis. The techniques of reduction and fixation depend on the patient, type and location of the fracture, associated injuries, and the experience of the surgeon. It should be remembered that an excellent result can be obtained in treatment of fractures without "anatomic" reduction of each fracture

fragment as long as the overall alignment of the bone is restored.

Reduction is either closed when functional alignment of the bone can be restored and fixation achieved without exposure of the fracture, or open when treatment cannot be achieved with closed techniques. Fixation devices are also divided by consideration of whether compression can be produced across the fragment surfaces or not. With adequate compression, movement is eliminated and callus formation is small, while in other fractures only support or "buttress" plating can be obtained and the callus formation may be rather large.

Screws

Screws convert torque into compression and are primarily used to provide interfragmental compression across a fracture site and to attach plates to bone. A screw that crosses a fracture line should be placed as a lag screw meaning that only the threads on the "far" fragment gain purchase (Fig. 4-85). These screws do not provide sufficient fixation to protect most fractures from the normal bending, rotation, and axial-loading forces encountered by the bone. These forces must be neutralized, usually by additional use of a plate. Multiple screws may be used to provide rotational stability.

Two basic types of screws are available, cortical and cancellous. Cortical screws are threaded over their entire length and usually have blunt ends with shallow threads that are closely spaced. They can be used as a lag screw. Cancellous screws have a wide thread diameter and a large area between threads to improve purchase of the screw in cancellous bone. They can be partially threaded and also serve as lag screws (Fig. 4-86). Special screws are hollow and are inserted over small-diameter guide pins, with pin removal after screw placement. Both cortical and cancellous screws are available as cannulated screws.

Radiographic examination of post-operative fractures should evaluate screw placement, especially the number of cortices that are engaged. The position of the fragments should be evaluated since the tighter the placement, the quicker the fracture healing. Screw placement can actually displace fracture fragments and hold them at a distance from other fragments. This needs to be identified, and hopefully corrected. On later radiographic studies, examination should include the identification of screws that are loosening, those that have pulled out of the bone, or those that have broken when subjected to excess loads. Screws in an infected environment show increased lucency within the bone around the screw, with localized pockets of osteolysis. If there is a generalized enveloping lucent zone around a screw, it is more likely due to movement of the screw without infection. Protruding screws can cause irritation to

the soft tissues, without any radiographic change except for soft tissue swelling.

Plates

Plates come in various sizes and shapes and function to compress, neutralize, or buttress. Compression plates are used in reduction and stabilization of fractures that are stable when placed in compression. However, these plates may also be used in combination with additional lag screws. Certain bones have a compression or tension side and a plate placed on the tension side absorbs the tensile forces, resulting in dynamic compression of the fracture. Neutralization plates only protect fracture surfaces from normal bending, rotation, and axial-loading forces and are often used in combination with lag screws which are usually placed separately from the plate (Fig. 4-85). Some plates both compress and neutralize the loading forces. Buttress plates support bone that is unstable under compression or axial loading, and are used for repairing fractures with severely comminuted fragments.

The plates may be straight with round holes or may have oval holes with inclined edges if they are to function as dynamic compression plates. Tubular plates are thin and have a concave inner surface that conforms to the curvature of the bone surface and are pliable and easier to contour. Contoured (Figs. 4-87, 4-88) or reconstruction plates are designed to allow bending, twisting, and contouring to accommodate bones with unusual shapes such as the acetabulum. Other special plates have a special shape such as a T- or L-shape.

In the repair of fractures, the use of plating alters both the manner of fracture healing and the way this appears radiographically. With minimal movement at the fracture site, callus formation is rather exuberant, being a good radiographic indicator of fracture healing that can be evaluated as to the time of its appearance and the amount of callus formed. With anatomic reduction and rigid fixation, the amount of callus formation is limited; the absence of this pattern of bone development on the radiograph may be of concern leading to a suspicion of non-healing. With these animals, evaluation of the fracture line on the radiographs is critical as its disappearance is an indication of healing.

Complications of plating include fatigue fractures as a result of excessive motion and repetitive stress; these occur in implants subjected to prolonged cyclic loading. Often, this is considered to be the result of a race between bone healing and fatigue failure of the plate. While a fractured plate is easily noticed radiographically (Fig. 4-89), it is important to evaluate the technique of original fixation since it may be possible to predict that there is insufficient stability to avoid cycling and subsequent plate fracture. Another problem results if the plate provides excessive support to the bone.

In this situation, the cortex beneath the plate becomes thin because there is no need for the bone tissue to support the limb. This kind of bone atrophy must be noted radiographically because it indicates the presence of weakened bone; this may result in a new fracture following removal of the plate when the original fracture has healed. Therefore, the originally fractured bone often needs some type of support following removal of stabilization devices until the bone regains original strength.

Osteomyelitis in the bone beneath the plate produces focal lucencies that are recognized only on a perfect lateral projection of the plate (radiographic projection underneath along the plate). The infection may also lead to loosening of the screws. Usually bone infection associated with fracture healing is suspected clinically prior to radiographic evidence of this complication.

Wires

K wires are unthreaded segments of extruded wire of variable thickness that are drilled into bone by placing them into a drill as if they were drill bits. Wires provide rotational stability when more than one is used (Fig. 4-90). K wires are also used for fixation of small bone fragments. They can be placed across the physeal plate without injury to the growth potential of the plate since they are smooth and the growing bone "slides" along the wire. K wires can also serve as guide pins for the placement of cannulated screws.

Cerclage wiring is a technique of placing a wire around the bone to stabilize fracture fragments; it is usually used in combination with other types of fixation devices (Figs. 4-91, 4-92) but can also be used alone. The radiographic examination must evaluate whether the wires are tightly positioned, since loose wires that move along the shaft of a bone disrupt the new periosteal blood supply that originates from the surrounding soft tissues. In this situation, frequently the end result will be a non-union fracture healing. A hemicerclage wire does not encircle the entire shaft but enters and exits through the cortex at one side (Fig. 4-93). Often, post-surgical control radiographs that are made to determine the progression of fracture healing reveal that cerclage wires have been broken. The significance of the broken wires depends on the development of the healing callus that stabilizes the fracture. If the fracture proves to be healed based on identification of a bridging callus, the presence of the broken wires is of little consequence. However, when fracture healing is only partially completed, the finding of broken wires is of great clinical significance since it indicates motion at the fracture site. Occasionally, post-surgical radiographs show that newly formed bone has grown over the wires making their removal difficult if not impossible (Fig. 4-91).

Tension-band wiring is a special orthopedic technique used to provide dynamic compression for the treatment of avulsion-type fractures, such as those involving the olecranon, tibial crest, or patella, or for the replacement of those apophyses that have to be removed surgically to provide access to a bone or joint. Parallel K wires are placed to provide rotational stability and reduce shearing forces between the fragments. A figure-of-eight wire is placed on the tension side of the bone and is anchored by passing it around both ends of the K wires and through a drilled hole in the bone (Figs. 4-64, 4-71). When physiological forces pull on the bone, the wire carries the tensile force, which prevents separation, transmitting compressive forces to the bone (Fig. 4-94). With time, the figure-of-eight wires may break or slip free due to bending of the straight wires. This is a problem only when it occurs early in the course of fracture healing. Tension-band wiring is rarely associated with an infectious process.

External fixation devices

External fixation is a technique in which individual bone fragments are held in place by percutaneous wires or pins attached to an external frame that may be metallic or synthetic. External fixation devices are versatile and allow for compression, neutralization, or distraction of fracture fragments, and some devices can even be adjusted in position over time to improve fragment reduction. They are often used for fractures associated with severe soft-tissue injury or contamination, to minimize the surgical trauma to the soft tissues while obtaining fragment fixation and stabilization. They may be used in special cases, such as bone lengthening, arthrodesis, fractures requiring distraction, infected fractures, and nonunion fractures. Some types have bars that connect the pins, others have rings that partially or completely surround the limb (Ilizarov), and others have a combination of clamps, bars, and rings.

Pins can be smooth or threaded and are referred to by a variety of names usually associated with the name of the inventor. Steinman pins are large-caliber wires with pointed tips that are cut to a desired length, and are used for fixation of fractures or for traction. Unilateral or one-half pins have threads at one end and enter the soft tissues on one side through a small skin incision and thread directly into the bone (Figs. 4-95, 4-96, 4-97).

Radiographic evaluation of these devices must include evaluation of the placement of the pins and ensure that both cortices of the bone shaft are penetrated. The entire bone needs to be included on the radiograph since the devices may be some distance from the fracture site. Penetration of the tip of a pin into soft tissues should be recognized and remedied since this can be a source of pain for the animal. External fixation is often used with complex injuries and complications are not uncommon. As the fracture heals, a regular lucency that envelops the pins where they pass through the cortices can be expected, and is the result of motion of the pins. Usually, it does not indicate an infectious process. Lucencies due to irregular areas of osteolysis are more suggestive of osteomyelitis. Pin-track infection is a frequent complication and is related to the technique of pin insertion, care of the pin site, and stresses on the pin-bone interface.

The location and position of the pins should be compared on subsequent radiographs as they may be forced out as a result of movement or infection. The pins may bend, especially if stress is placed across the fracture site; however, since they do not cycle, they rarely break.

Intramedullary fixation devices
Intramedullary devices can be solid or hollow, circular, triangular, or cloverleaf in cross section; they can be flexible to rigid, and can be placed in reamed or unreamed channels. Most pins are hollow and almost all have a specific cross-sectional pattern designed to reduce or prevent rotation. The terms rod, nail, and pin have specific biomechanical implications, but clinically the names are used interchangeably. The devices can be used singularly or stacked (more than one). Radio-ulnar fractures are often stabilized using intramedullary pinning (Fig. 4-98). It is common practice to use an intramedullary pin in conjunction with another fixation device (Figs. 4-91, 4-96).

Radiographs made to evaluate fracture healing stabilized with intramedullary devices show the fracture with a preponderance of extracortical callus, since most of the medullary blood supply has been destroyed by the original injury and the subsequent reaming procedure prevents formation of intramedullary callus until a later time. Often the fragments of a long bone tend to telescope around the pin, with resultant shortening of the bone and additional fragmentation at the original fracture site. Rotation of the fragments may occur if axial stability has not been achieved using other techniques and the relationship of the ends of the bone must be examined to evaluate this. It is not uncommon for the proximal femoral fragment to rotate into a position that results in anteversion of the femoral head. The original fracture needs to be carefully examined to ascertain the presence or absence of long fissure fracture(s) in addition to the more transverse fracture, since this may result in additional fractures during the placement of the pins. Detection of these additional fissure fracture lines should discourage the use of an intramedullary pin for fixation. In smaller animals, the pins may migrate and protrude through the end of a bone into the joint space or into adjacent soft tissues.

Placement of intramedullary pins across a physeal growth plate is acceptable only if they are smooth. A threaded pin holds the cancellous bone both proximally and distally to the growth plate and results in compression of the physeal plate with consequent premature closure and prevention of bone growth. Even so, pins cannot be placed in a crossing manner across a growth plate since this also results in premature closure of the growth plate and delayed growth. Sometimes pins are placed across a joint space with the end of the pin entering the opposing bone preventing motion of the joint. This is acceptable for a limited period of time with the knowledge that soft tissues contract and get rigid ultimately preventing normal range of motion following removal of the pin. Pins should not be placed in a way that the tip enters the joint space while the opposing bone can still move since this will cause severe injury to the articular surface due to the gouging action of the tip of the pin. All of these points must be evaluated radiographically.

Lucency may be noted around the pins during healing. Because of the way in which these pins are placed, most of the shaft of the pin is within the medullary cavity; an infectious process resulting in destruction of the surrounding cancellous bone post-operatively can be almost impossible to identify. If the osteolysis is focal in location and periosteal new bone forms adjacent to the suspect lesion, osteomyelitis should be suspected. Radiolucency at points of contact with the endosteal surface could be due to motion or bone infection.

4. Joint Injury

Instability of a joint can be referred to as luxation, subluxation, or dislocation depending on the degree of instability and separation of the articular surfaces. Detection of injury to the joints is quite easily seen in most traumatized animals, although the radiographic evaluation is dependent on the anatomical features of the joint involved. Unfortunately, positioning of the limb for the radiographic study may reduce any luxation or instability and cause the joint to appear nearly normal. Stress studies are therefore necessary to fully appreciate radiographically the degree of luxation or instability. It is important to understand that strain or sprain of the soft tissues surrounding a joint often require a much longer time for healing than does a fracture, where the major injury is to bone tissue. The manner in which a joint injury heals is greatly affected by the degree of successful reduction of the luxation and by the maintenance of the normal anatomical alignment of the bones during the time of soft tissue repair.

4.1. Anatomical location
Shoulder joint
The shoulder is anatomically unique in that there are no definite ligaments that maintain humeral head and glenoid cavity in persistent position. Consequently, on

radiographs made with abduction or traction, the joint space appears to increase in width, suggesting luxation. In some patients, it is difficult to determine whether a chronic luxation is post-traumatic or congenital (Figs. 4-99, 4-100).

Elbow joint
The elbow joint is relatively easy to evaluate radiographically because it is a tightly fitting joint and luxation results in marked separation of the ends of the bones, with or without associated fractures (Fig. 4-101).

Carpal and phalangeal joints
Injury to the antebracheocarpal, intercarpal, and carpometacarpal joints is best evaluated on hyperextended or other stress views that demonstrate the degree of ligamentous injury and associated fractures, and the resulting joint laxity in the best manner. In animals with injury to the collateral ligaments, stress views can be made with the foot forced into a valgus or varus position (Fig. 4-102). Interphalangeal joints are more difficult to evaluate radiographically and it may be necessary to force the foot into contact with the cassette using a plastic or wooden paddle.

Hip joint
The hip joint is relatively easy to evaluate post-traumatically since the femoral head tends to separate completely from the acetabulum and luxate to a position dorsocranially alongside the ilium. It is important to examine the radiograph for associated acetabular fractures (Fig. 4-103). A difficulty in diagnosis occurs in the animal in which the acute trauma is superimposed over a dysplastic hip joint that was previously unstable due to joint capsule stretching and flattening of the acetabular cup. The same problem occurs with a luxation detected in an animal with chronic changes following aseptic necrosis of the femoral head (Fig. 4-79). If the animal is in pain during the radiographic procedure, it is possible to make the study with the legs in a fully flexed position.

Stifle joint
The stifle joint is more difficult to evaluate radiographically, compared with joints that have articular surfaces that are more congruent, such as the elbow or hip. In tightly fitting joints, the components are either "in" or "out" and diagnosis of injury is easier. Because the joint space between the "round" femoral condyles and the "flattened" tibial plateau changes in width, it is difficult to understand what is normal radiographically. These bones "fit" only because of the radiographically invisible menisci. Therefore, luxation of the stifle joint is more difficult to ascertain radiographically, although it is possible to attempt to generate cranial displacement of the tibia or separation of the bones using stress techniques (Fig. 4-104). Application of craniocaudal stress may demonstrate cruciate ligament injury, while application of mediolateral stress may demonstrate collateral ligament injury.

Tarsus and phalangeal joints
The tibiotarsal joint is a tightly fitting joint. Instability usually results from fracture of one of the malleoli, with resulting luxation that is easily seen on the radiographs (Fig. 4-105). Injury to this joint may be better visualized radiographically by stressing the foot into valgus or varus positions. Intertarsal and tarsometatarsal joints usually require stress radiographs to fully evaluate the degree of joint instability and associated fractures (Fig. 4-106). The tarsometatarsal joint is best evaluated in hyperflexed and hyperextended positions. If the injury is extensive enough, the bones remain permanently malpositioned (Fig. 4-107).

4.2. Other traumatically induced joint diseases
Intra-articular fractures
Fractures that enter the joint space disrupt the articular cartilage; as a result, the healing process leaves a roughened or irregular articular surface (Figs. 4-37, 4-38, 4-39, 4-49, 4-60, 4-62, 4-64, 4-86). This irregularity of the cartilaginous surface undergoes remodelling with development of a secondary arthrosis. The degree of original injury to the joint surface plus the level of anatomic restoration determines the degree of arthrosis that will develop (Fig. 4-108). Features such as the size and weight of the animal, and the degree of daily/weekly exercise, also determine the level of the resulting arthrosis. It is important that the clinician understands this concept because it makes it possible to forewarn the owner that a fracture/luxation which is repaired and seems to be healing without acute complications may cause secondary changes of long-lasting clinical significance.

Fracture-luxation
Fracture-luxation is a combination of injury to the bone as well as injury to the joint. The fracture may be intra-articular or extra-articular. The clinical significance of articular fractures is greater and more severe if reduction of the luxation and repositioning of intra-articular bony fragments does not result in restoration of a normal anatomical relationship. Any resulting instability or malalignment of the joint surface leads to development of post-traumatic arthrosis. Injury of this type is more important in a heavy, athletic animal when it concerns an important weight-bearing joint. If the fracture is extra-articular, the avulsion of the tendinous and ligamentous attachments may not be appreciated and the lesion undertreated (Fig .4-109).

Hemarthrosis
The immediate results of the crushing of the synovial membrane of a joint or its communicating bursa are hemorrhage and edema. The amount of fluid produced is large, and out of proportion to the injury, although this transudate is usually

absorbed within a few days. However, if the injury is more violent, blood may collect within the joint space interrupting the nutrition of the articular cartilage. In the event of underlying blood dyscrasias such as hemophilia, the resulting bleeding may be exaggerated following a rather minor trauma. Hemarthrosis is recognized radiographically by distension of the joint capsule; the character of the intra-articular fluid can only be known following arthrocentesis. Hemarthrosis is an uncommon clinical finding following trauma in animals. It is not as important in animals as it is in man, where patients with hemophilia frequently have bleeding diathesis.

Chronic joint disease

An animal with chronic joint disease often demonstrates acute lameness and a level of pain that is unexpected considering the nature of the injury that has been sustained. As a result, a dog or cat following rather minimal trauma may have a non-weight-bearing lameness. The reason for this becomes obvious when chronic arthrosis is detected radiographically (Fig. 4-110). The purpose of a radiographic examination is to determine the cause of pain so that other lesions of an acute nature requiring fixation and stabilization can be excluded. Often, more chronic injuries have already resulted in the formation of pseudoarthrosis (Fig. 4-111)

Joint bodies

Joint bodies by definition are detached fragments within a joint that result from acute trauma or a degenerative change that is often related to an antecedental traumatic episode. The position of the joint bodies may remain fixed or may change causing various clinical signs. As they are maybe made of bony tissue and have increased tissue density, they are frequently noted radiographically. However, it is often difficult to determine their origin or the degree of freedom of movement. Etiologies for these little, dense bodies are multiple and include: (1) avulsion fracture fragments, (2) synovial osteochondromas, (3) areas of chronic dystrophic calcification within the joint capsule, (4) calcified menisci, or (5) calcified osteochondral fragments.

Sometimes, the location of the dense body is diagnostic of its etiology. An example of this is the joint body that can be found in the stifle joint due to avulsion of a small fragment of bone at the attachment site of the cranial cruciate ligament on the tibial plateau (Fig. 4-112). A body resting in the caudal pouch of the shoulder joint in a dog with humeral head osteochondrosis usually results from a separated osteochondral fragment. Avulsion fractures from the acetabular rim may be found within the depth of the acetabular cup and make reduction of the luxation of the femoral head difficult (Fig. 4-103). Bony or cartilaginous bodies within the joint often attach to the reactive synovium, develop a blood supply, and mature with time into larger, more amorphous appearing bodies. In ani-

mals, it is very uncommon that these joint bodies move freely through the affected joint, as is seen in the knee of humans where osteochondral fragments move between articular surfaces, become trapped, and cause acute pain. In animals, it is more likely that the bodies are attached and cause a chronic synovitis that is painful. However, one common exception to this rule is the shoulder pain that results from fragmentation of a large osteochondral flap from the humeral head when the fragments move cranially and distally and become lodged inside the tendon sheat around the tendon of the biceps brachi muscle.

Intra-articular gas

Curvilinear or streaky radiolucent shadows within a joint are due to the presence of gas, usually air. The shadows may be present following a compound injury in which air gains direct access to the joint. More commonly, the presence of the gas follows a diagnostic arthrocentesis. Rarely is the gas directly related to the presence of gas-producing organisms. It is possible to find gas outlining a joint surface when the resultant traumatic forces are so directed that they pull the articular cartilages apart and create a vacuum phenomenon. This phenomenon, which is due to the accumulation of nitrogen gas that comes from the synovial blood-vessels, is commonly present in radiographs of the shoulder joint of dogs when made with traction, especially in the presence of cartilage lesions.

Post-traumatic septic arthritis

While septic arthritis following trauma is common in foals and calves, post-traumatic joint infection in small animals is uncommon and occurs most of the time in association with bite wounds in cats. The condition may also follow joint surgery. The first radiographic changes that are, however, non-specific are those of soft tissue swelling with capsular distension. Later, the subchondral bone becomes osteopenic and a fluffy pattern of periosteal new bone is seen equally distributed on both sides of the joint. The infection may occur in a joint in which there is pre-existing secondary joint disease in which there are lytic changes in the form of distinct subchondral bone cysts or a generalized osteopenia. Any new bone lysis as a result of the septic arthritis may therefore be difficult to identify because of the superimposition of the new lysis over destructive changes already present. New bone production may also be lost within the periarticular enthesophyte formations belonging to the already existing deformative arthrosis. The infection is usually detected clinically before the radiographic signs are conclusive (Fig. 4-113). In an animal with chronic infectious joint disease, the radiographic changes may include destruction of large portions of adjacent bones, with marked distortion of articular surfaces (Fig. 4-114). Septic joints that are chronic may have associated soft tissue atrophy that makes dislocation possible.

Neurotrophic joints

Neurotrophic arthropathies include those associated with syringomyelia or other neurologic diseases in which the intact sense of balance and pain that is essential for the preservation of joint integrity has been removed subjecting the joint to persistent misuse and chronic trauma. This type of joint disease in animals is uncommon, and is largely associated with sectioning of a nerve as a treatment for a chronic orthopedic disease such as navicular disease in horses.

5. Pathological Fractures

Pathological fractures of the spine

Pathological fractures are uncommon in animals and may involve a single bone or multiple bones and may be due to malignant disease, or more commonly, due to nutritional disease. These fractures are often not complete, but instead are of a "folding" or "bending" pattern. In the spine, the fractured vertebral bodies are of a compression type with the ventral cortex "folded" (Fig. 4-115). Radiographic diagnosis is usually made by noting shortened vertebral bodies with a thinner vertebral end-plate and preserved disc spaces. The shortening of the vertebral bodies often creates a kyphosis or scoliosis. The abnormal vertebrae are most easily seen on lateral views in the lumbar region because of the absence of overlying bony shadows. Ventrodorsal or dorsoventral views are usually not helpful because of overlying soft tissue shadows. The density of the bony segments may be less than normal but this may be difficult to determine from the radiograph.

Multiple fractures are often associated with secondary nutritional hyperparathyroidism in a younger animal on an unbalanced diet. Bone density in these rapidly growing animals is minimal even under the best nutritional conditions, and the determination of what is pathological is difficult. One test that can be used is the examination of the radiographic presentation of the ventral cortex of the vertebral bodies. Normally, the cortex is represented by rather sharply defined dense lines that contrast with the less dense cancellous bone in the vertebral body and the less dense perivertebral soft tissues. If this line is missing, it is an indicator of osteopenia.

Pathological fractures of the mandible

Pathological fractures in the mandible are usually associated with renal osteodystrophy that results in a remarkable degree of osteopenia. The same loss of bone density is seen in the maxilla and premaxilla, but fractures are less common. Pathological fractures in the mandible may also be associated with chronic periodontal disease.

Pathological fractures of long bones

Pathological fractures in long bones are usually multiple, due to nutritional problems, and are most easily detected by the abnormal conformation of the bones. At the site of fracture, bending or folding cortices cause an increased bone density due to the "doubling" of the cortical bone (Fig. 4-116). Careful examination of other bones may reveal additional fractures, sometimes of older duration and healed (Fig. 4-117). The bended cortical shadows that are present with acute fractures repair with an uneven thickness of the new cortical lining. In addition, on the concave side there is a generalized increased thickness of the cortex where it is strengthened because of greater weight-bearing.

Pathological fractures in long bones may also be associated with a solitary bone lesion such as a benign bone cyst, or with a malignant bone lesion such as a primary bone tumor (Fig. 4-118). With every fracture, it is important to closely evaluate the character of the surrounding bony tissue to ascertain that the fracture does not involve diseased bone.

6. Soft Tissue Trauma

Radiographs seldom play a role in evaluation of isolated soft tissue injuries unless there is a question of retained foreign material. Lacerations may cause accumulation of gas within the soft tissues making radiographic evaluation more difficult. When large portions of skin and underlying muscle, tendon, and ligaments are removed as is seen with abrasive injuries, the radiographic evaluation should include a description of the highly significant soft tissue injury.

Soft tissue swelling

Soft tissue swelling is difficult to detect on radiographs of the axial skeleton or proximal portions of the limbs, and is more easily seen around the feet distally. When detected, soft tissue swelling is a good indicator of the location of the injury. A good rule is to permit the soft tissue swelling to direct the attention to the lesion in the underlying bone (Figs. 4-119, 4-120). If a bony lesion is present, it is often in this location.

In the absence of instability or fracture, swollen joints are often associated with strain or sprain. Unfortunately, it is not always appreciated that soft tissue injuries are slowly healing, and, for that reason, may be more significant than a fracture.

Soft tissue gas

Gas within soft tissues is commonly seen in trauma cases when the integrity of the skin has been broken. Air accumulates in the subcutaneous tissues and/or may follow the muscle bellies. When it is not convenient to physically examine a fractured limb, identification of the gas on the radiograph is the first indication of the open nature of the fracture. Also post-surgically, gas may be present in the soft tissues. (Figs. 4-85, 4-121). It is possible, but very uncommon, that the gas in the soft tissues is the result of an infection by a gas-producing organism. If that is the case, the gas more commonly assumes a pattern of small bubbles equally spread throughout the diseased tissues.

Soft tissue radiopacity
Any radiopacity within the soft tissues is suggestive of a penetrating foreign body and has significance. Careful evaluation should also be directed to discern an additional underlying bone injury (Fig. 4-122). Areas of calcification within the soft tissues are indicative of chronic injury and are not associated with an acute injury (Fig.4-123). The exact location within the body of a single radiopacity seen radiographically may be settled by drawing a cross-section picture of the body and locating the planes within which the foreign body lies as determined from both orthogonal views. The intersection of these planes along with the location in a proximal-distal direction, specifically locates the foreign body. If further localization is required, it is possible to place radiopaque skin markers and make additional radiographic exposures. It is also possible to insert radiopaque needles into the soft tissues to provide markers to be used during surgical exploration.

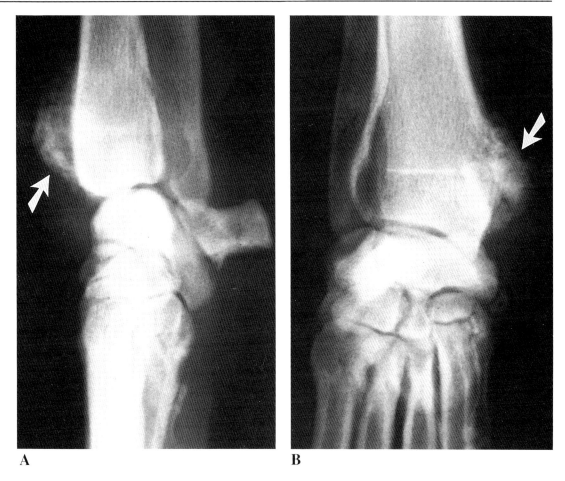

A   B

Figure 4-1.
Post-traumatic enthesophyte formation.
*The focal increase in bone tissue on the medial (**A**) and cranial (**B**) aspect of the distal radius is due to periosteal new bone formation secondary to trauma, 1 month previously. Tearing of ligamentous attachments, or entheses, often results in this type of new bone production, referred to as an enthesophyte (arrows). Note that the joint spaces are unaffected and that the subchondral bone has remained normal in appearance. The dog was 6 months of age at the time of injury and soft tissue attachments to bone were loose, partially explaining the exuberance of the new bone response.*

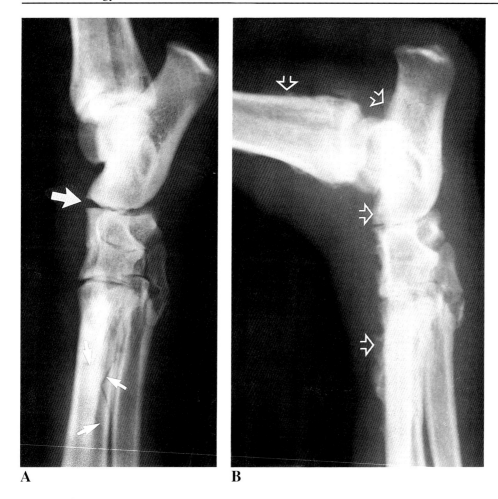

A   B

Figure 4-2.
Post-traumatic enthesophyte formation.
*A 6-year-old male German Shepherd Dog sustained an acute dislocation of the proximal intertarsal joint (**A**, large arrow). The instability at the site of injury was demonstrated with a lateral view of the foot, made with the digits stressed into a hyperflexed position. Fractures of the third metatarsal bone were also present (A, small arrows).*
*A second radiograph (**B**), made 8 weeks post-injury, showed areas of increased periosteal new bone (hollow arrows) due to the tearing of the ligamentous and tendinous attachments around the joints. While this response was rather prominent in this patient, it may be even more exuberant in a younger patient in which the soft tissues are more loosely attached to the bone. The presence of the periosteal response as seen in this case can be expected following trauma to the limb; however, a similar pattern of periosteal response is also expected in a patient with a post-traumatic infectious arthritis or osteomyelitis. Physical examination is important in making the differentiation.*
In this patient, the soft tissue swelling was hard, firm, and not warm; the foot was not painful, and it was not possible to aspirate fluid from the affected joints. These findings are supportive of the idea that the new bone formation was post-traumatic in nature and not infectious.

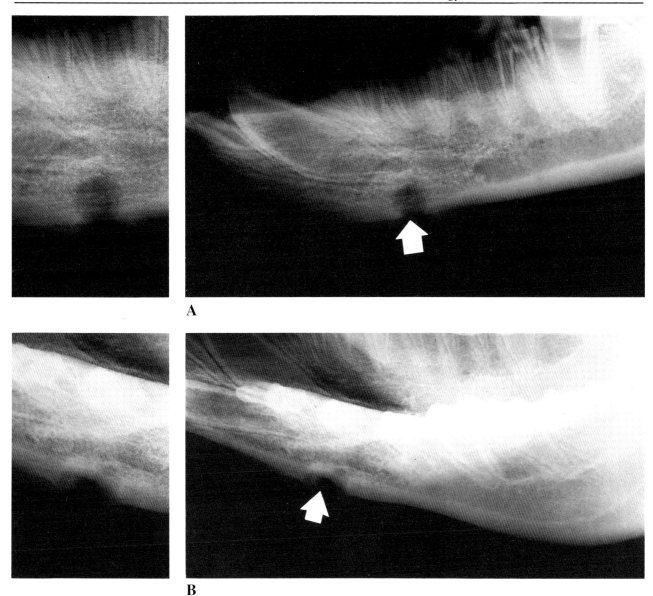

A

B

Figure 4-3.
Post-traumatic periosteal new bone formation.
*A 6-month-old female Irish Wolfhound had a hard swollen lesion on the right mandible at the level of first premolar teeth, first noticed 12 days earlier and increasing in size since that time. On lateral (**A**) and oblique (**B**) radiographs of the mandible, a discrete destructive lesion with surrounding reactive periosteal new bone was seen (arrows). Periosteal new bone formation of this type is often associated with a forgotten rubber band that had been placed around the lower jaw. The biopsy report of the bony tissue indicated that the periosteal response was compatible with chronic irritation by a foreign body without evidence of osteomyelitis.*

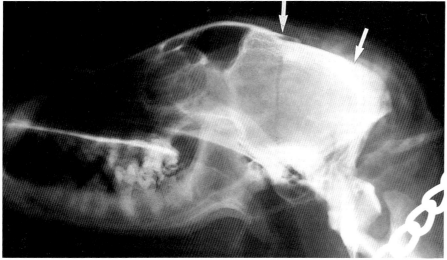

A

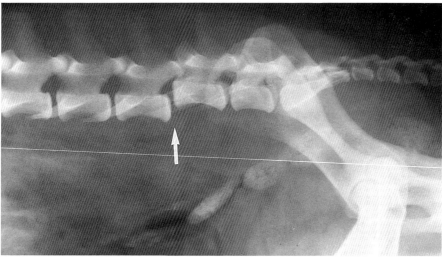

B

Figure 4-4.
Skull and spinal fractures.

*This 4-year-old male Terrier-cross was presented after being hit by a car several hours earlier. The dog was moribund at the time of presentation and a neurological examination could not be adequately performed. A lateral view of the head (**A**) demonstrated fracture lines through the temporal and parietal bones (arrows), while a lateral view of the spine (**B**) demonstrated a fracture-luxation at L5-6 (arrow). This is an example of a survey radiographic study on a seriously injured patient for the purpose of determining the full extent of the present injuries. The dog died two days later.*

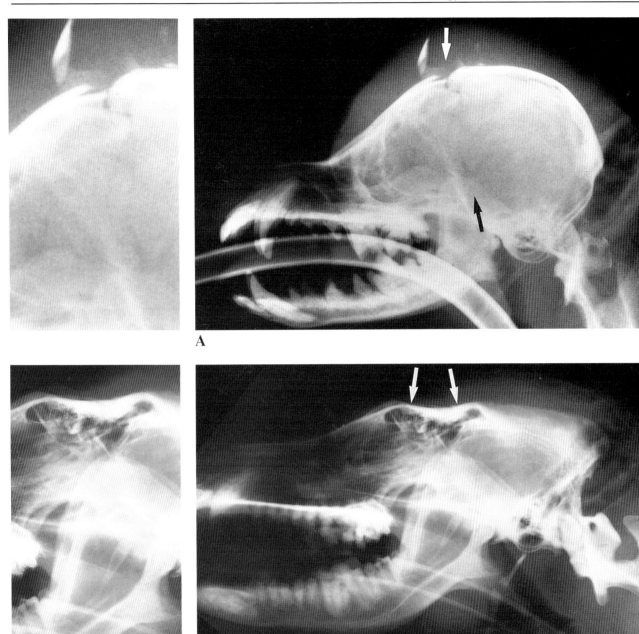

Figure 4-5.
Skull fractures.
Lateral radiographs of the head of a 4-year-old Terrier-cross (A) that was hit by a car shortly before presentation and of the head of an 8-year-old German Shepherd Dog that worked for a Police Department (B) that was hit by a car 6 to 8 months previously. These two studies show the differences in conformation of the head dependent on breed and how trauma can be expressed differently on the radiograph.

The first dog (A) was brought to the clinic shortly after the accident when she was in a coma, hyperventilating, and showing intermittent decerebrate rigidity. Radiographs of the skull showed fractures of the frontal and temporal bones, with fracture lines extending to the basilar region of the skull (arrows). Note the marked soft tissue swelling over the frontal region of the head. Within the next few hours the dog became persistently decerebrate, developed respiratory paralysis, and died.

The second dog (B) developed exophthalmus of the left eye with congestion of the scleral and conjunctival vessels and protrusion of the third eyelid. The depression of bony fragments of the frontal bone into the frontal sinus is evident (arrows). This is an example of an extensive head trauma presenting few signs of damage to the central nervous system except for those affecting vision.

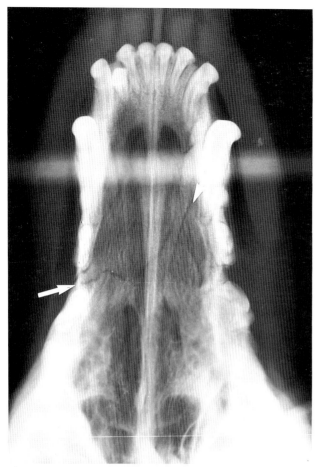

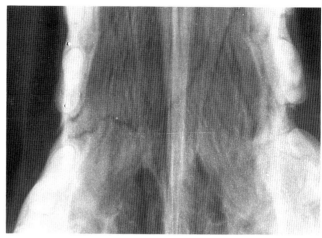

A

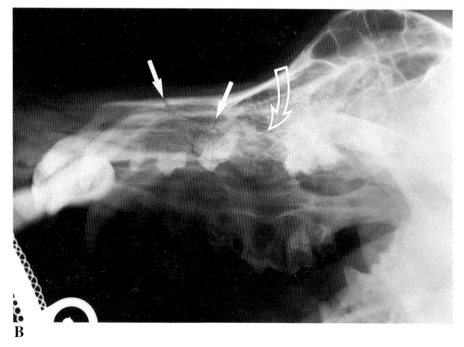

B

Figure 4-6.
Maxillary fractures.
Open mouth (A) and oblique (B) radiographs were made of the nasal region of a 1-year-old female Irish Setter. The dog had been hit by a car 4 days earlier and had developed epistaxis and progressive dyspnea. Fracture lines extend through the maxillary bones (solid arrows) without causing fragment displacement. The left fourth upper premolar has been lost (hollow arrow).

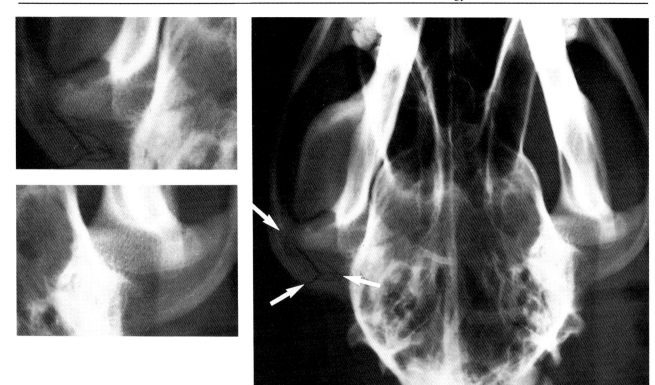

A

Figure 4-7.
Fractures of the zygomatic arch.
Ventrodorsal (A) and oblique (B) views of the head were made of this 10-year-old male Golden Retriever after it was struck by a car. The fracture lines involve the zygomatic arch and enter the temporo-mandibular joints (arrows). Fractures of this type heal well and the secondary post-traumatic joint disease is usually not a clinical problem.

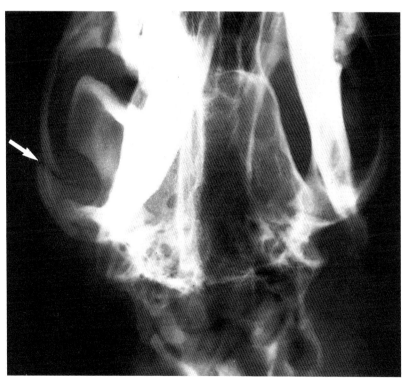

B

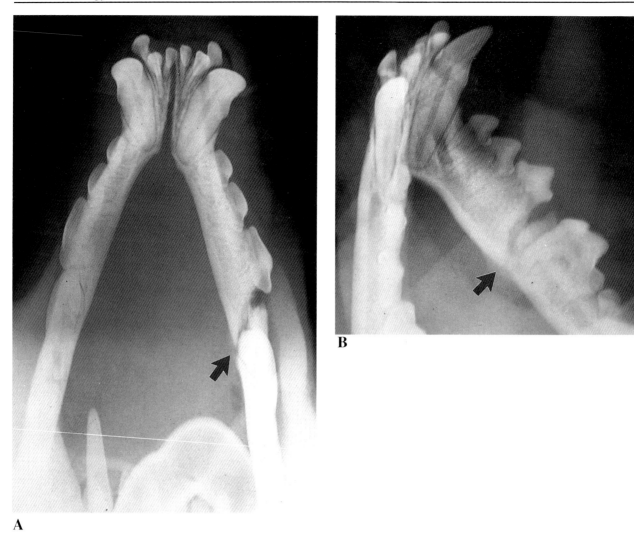

A

B

Figure 4-8.
Mandibular body fracture.
Radiographs of the mandible of a 2-year-old male Shih Tzu showed a transversely directed fracture between the 3rd and 4th lower premolars. Fracture lines entered the periodontal space of the 4th premolar (arrows). The study illustrates the value of the use of open-mouth radiographic technique.

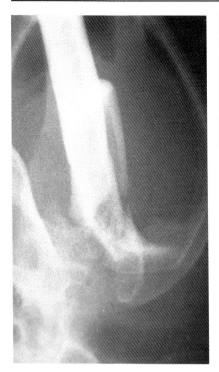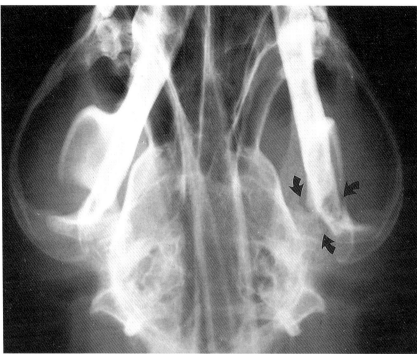

Figure 4-9.
Mandibular ramus fracture.
A 3-year-old male Samoyed was hit by a car 4 days earlier and was unable to eat normally after the injury. Radiographs of the head showed a comminuted fracture of the ramus and condylar process of the left mandible (arrows). These fractures are difficult to evaluate from a single radiograph, and it is usually helpful to use multiple radiographic views.

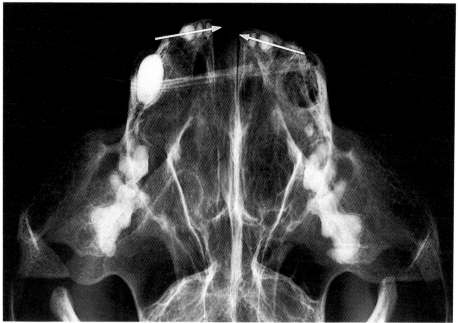

A

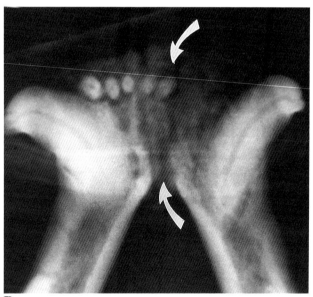

B

Figure 4-10.
Symphyseal fractures.
*A 14-year-old male cat presented with soft tissue swelling of unknown origin around the head. The open-mouth radiograph of the maxilla (**A**) demonstrated the malalignment of the incisor teeth (arrows) secondary to fractures of the palatine process of the incisive bone. Note the absence of the left canine and both first premolar teeth. The intra-oral radiograph of the mandibular symphyseal region (**B**) demonstrated another fracture line (arrows) extending from the symphysis to the middle incisor tooth on the left. Fracture lines within cancellous bone are not as clearly identified as those involving cortical bone. The radiograph lacks detail because of the use of radiographic magnification technique.*

Figure 4-11.
Dental fracture.
*Intra-oral (**A**) and oblique (**B**) radiographs were made of a 1-year-old female Lhasa Apso who was hit by a car. The right upper canine tooth was apparently fractured (large arrows) below the gingival attachment and the remaining root was fractured. A piece of crown was missing from the 3rd right upper incisor (small arrow). A part of the right premaxilla was fractured free (long arrows), and that part of the bone in which the incisors were imbedded was displaced rostrally.*

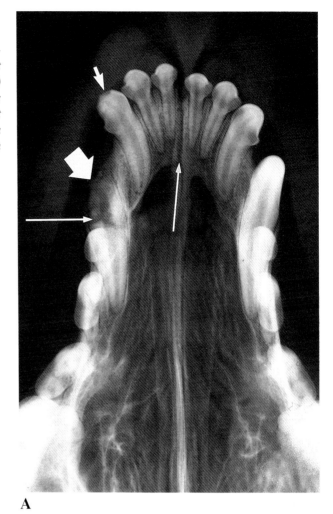

A

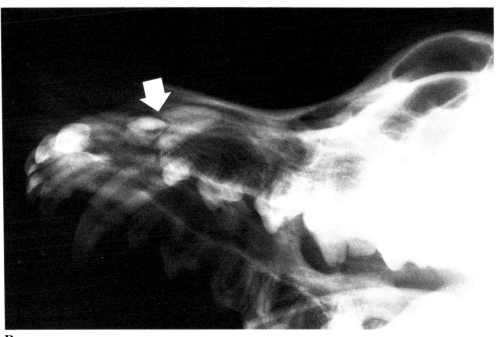

B

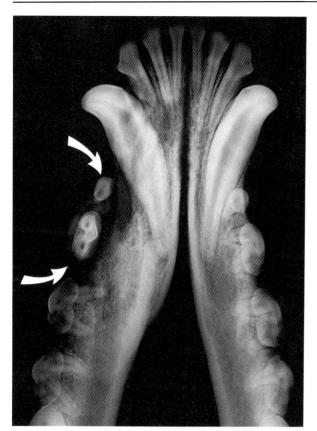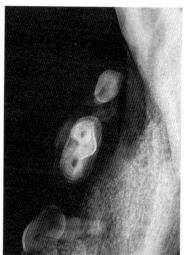

Figure 4-12.
Significance of dental or periodontal injury.
A 1-year-old male Golden Retriever had fractured the body of the mandible 7 weeks earlier, and was treated by pin placement through the medullary cavity of the mandible. The pin was removed 6 weeks after placement. The owner noted ulceration of the gum with visible bone tissue. A sequestrum (arrows) containing the 1st and 2nd lower premolars was identified on the intra-oral radiograph and was subsequently removed surgically.

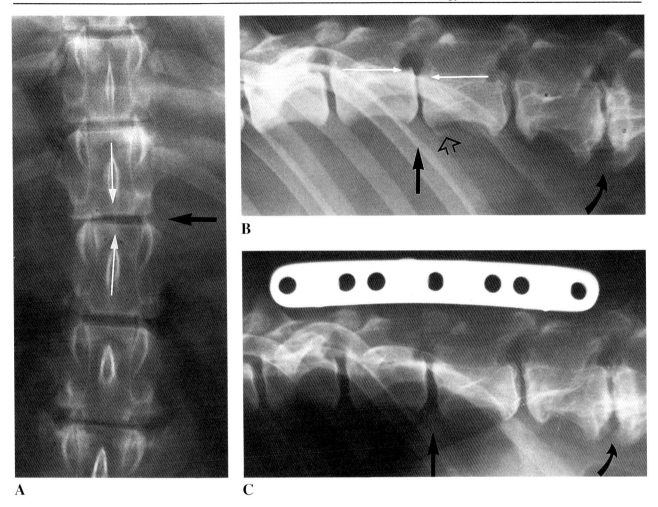

A **B** **C**

Figure 4-13.
Vertebral luxation.
*A 9-year-old spayed female Dalmation-mix was hit by a car 2 weeks earlier and was nonambulatory since the time of injury. Upper-motor neuron signs in the rear limbs were present, with good perception of deep pain. The radiographs showed malalignment of the vertebrae between T13 - L1 (**A**, straight white arrows). Notice the collapsed disc space at T13-L1, with uneven width (**B**, straight black arrows). A small fracture fragment from the body of L1 is displaced ventrally (B, hollow arrow).*
*An effort was made to stabilize the fracture/luxation with a dorsally positioned plate following decompressive hemilaminectomy (**C**). The disc space between L3-4 is partially collapsed but there is sclerosis of the endplates and vertebral spondylosis ventrally (black curved arrows) indicating that this is an old lesion and should not mistakenly be considered as the cause of the acute clinical signs.*

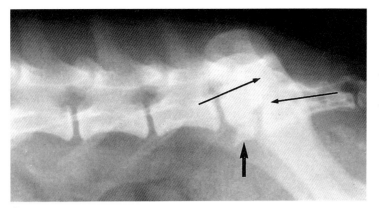

A

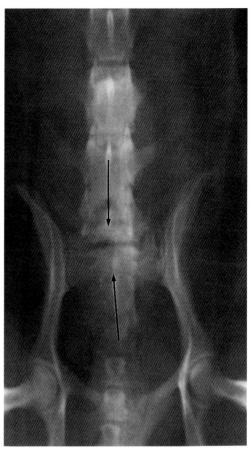

Figure 4-14.
Lumbosacral fracture-luxation.
A mature male small Terrier-cross returned home with paralysis of the tail and decreased anal sphincter tone. A fracture-luxation at the lumbosacral region with ventral displacement of the caudal sacral segment was noted on the radiographs. Malalignment of the floor of the spinal canal was identified (A, long arrows). In addition, a single large fracture fragment from the body of L7 that was displaced ventrally (A, large arrow) was also identified. Close examination of the spinous processes on the ventrodorsal view showed minimal displacement of the caudal fragment to the left (B, long arrows). It is convenient to use the alignment of these processes to evaluate traumatic displacement.

B

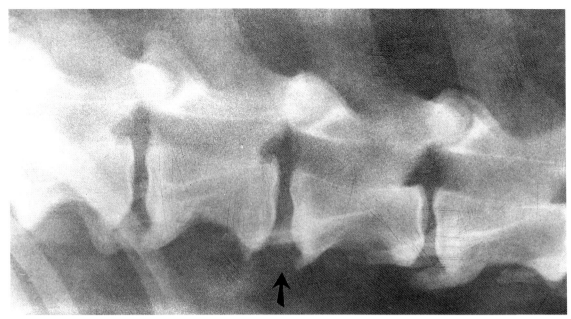

A

Figure 4-15.
Vertebral fracture-luxation.

Lateral (**A**) *and ventrodorsal* (**B**) *radiographs were made of the lumbar spine of a 6-year-old female Shepherd-cross that was injured one day earlier. Neurologic examination suggested an upper motor neuron lesion in the pelvic limbs. Notice the ease of identification of the fracture-luxation at L2-3 on the ventrodorsal view (B, large arrow) due to the lateral angulation and rotational instability. The same disc space on the lateral radiograph appeared normal or only slightly widened (A, arrow). The injury to the dorsal articular facets that permitted the instability was difficult to evaluate because of the underlying soft tissues shadows within the abdomen. The dorsal processes are visible (B, long arrows) and are rotated and angulated at the site of the injury. It is imperative that two orthogonal views be made on each patient.*

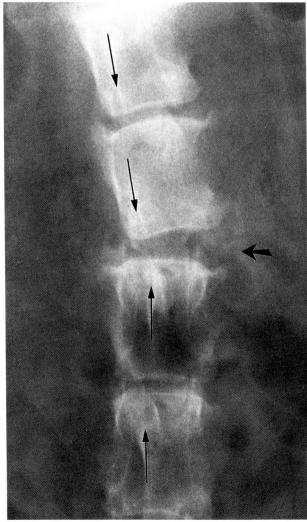

B

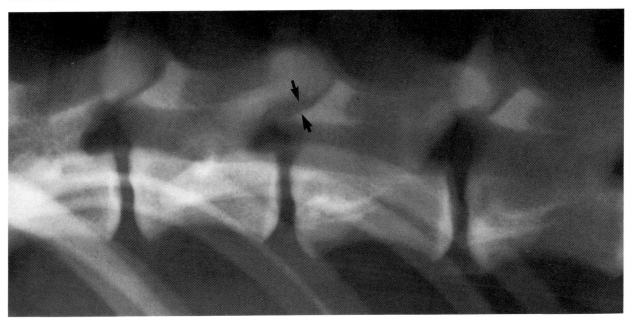

A

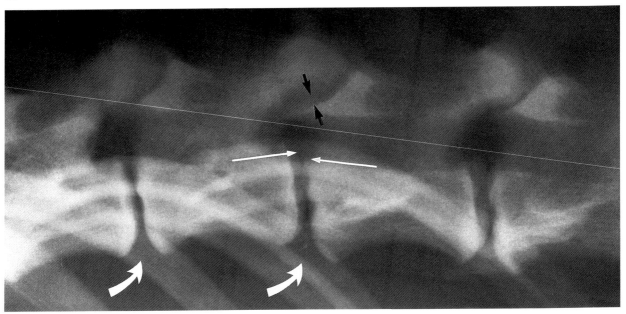

B

Figure 4-16.

Vertebral luxation.

Lateral spinal radiographs were made of a 3-year-old castrated male German Shepherd Dog, 20 days after a dog-fight. Since the fight, the dog had been persistently paretic in the fore limbs and paralyzed in the pelvic limbs. He had recovered some proprioceptive ability in the previous few days, but a deficiency remained. Patellar reflexes remained exaggerated. The radiograph made on the day of hospitalization (A) showed a near-normal appearance of the spine, with only an increase in width of the joint space of the true vertebral joints of T13-L1 (black arrows). The radiograph made 17 days later (B) continued to show the joint laxity dorsally (black arrows), but, in addition, showed instability of the disc with malalignment of the adjacent vertebral segments (long white arrows). Notice that both T12-13 and T13-L1 disc spaces are now narrowed (white curved arrows).

This is an example of a traumatic luxation of one and, possibly, two intervertebral discs with separation of the dorsal articular facets. The possibility of associated vertebral fractures cannot be excluded. A myelographic examination is necessary to learn more of the severity of the cord injury. Notice how the shadows cast by the ribs make radiographic evaluation of disc space width difficult.

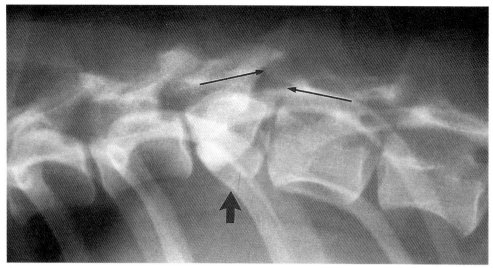

A

Figure 4-17.
Compression vertebral fracture.
Lateral (A) and ventrodorsal (B) radiographs were made of a 1-year-old male mixed-breed dog, injured 10 days earlier. The dog was paraplegic, had upper motor neuron signs in the hind limbs, but had a good deep pain sensation. The body of T12 was collapsed as seen on both views (thick arrows). The caudal portion of the T12 vertebral segment was displaced ventrally as seen by examination of the dorsal roof of the spinal canal (A, long arrows) and was displaced to the left as seen on the ventrodorsal radiograph (B, long arrows). This is an example of a rather severe vertebral fracture that did not result in severe injury to the spinal cord.

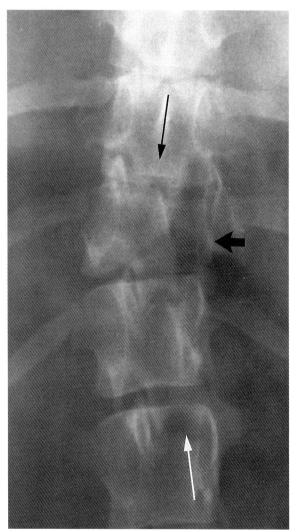

B

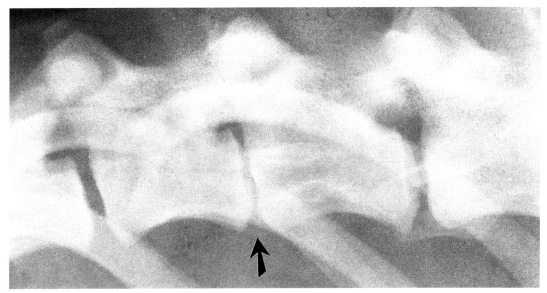

A

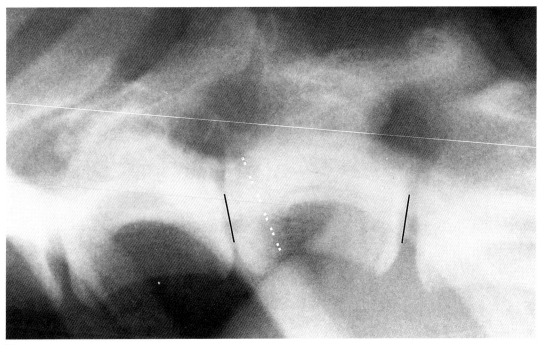

B

Figure 4-18.
Compression vertebral fracture.
*Lateral spinal radiographs made following trauma illustrate how the intervertebral disc can be involved in the injury in addition to the vertebral body. An 8-month-old female Irish Setter (**A**) presented with hyperrigidity of all four limbs. The radiographic signs were limited to collapse of the intervertebral disc space at T13-L1 (arrow). In another patient (**B**), collapse of a disc space was seen along with marked shortening of the vertebral body due to a compression fracture. The endplates were not parallel (black lines) and the fracture lines through the vertebral body were poorly identified (white dotted line).*

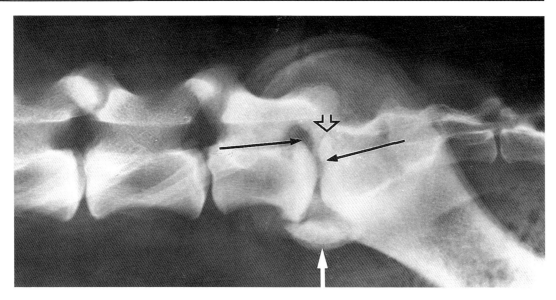

Figure 4-19.
Osteochondrosis of the sacrum.
Malalignment of the last lumbar vertebral body and the sacrum (long black arrows) with marked productive bony changes (white arrow) was associated with disc degeneration. Notice the diagnostically important small bony fragment that originates from the dorsal portion of the sacral endplate that is indicative of an osteochondral-type lesion (hollow arrow). This developmental lesion can lead to severe lumbosacral disc degeneration that ultimately leads to a cauda equine syndrome. Trauma to this unstable lumbosacral disc was thought to be the cause of the acute onset of neurologic signs in this dog.

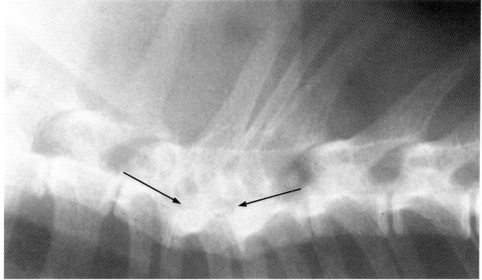

A

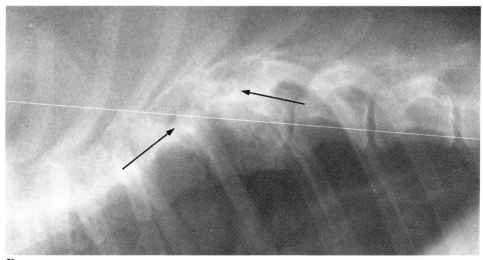

B

Figure 4-20.
Vertebral malalignment.

*Two patients with severe vertebral segment malalignment. Midthoracic lordosis was seen in a 2-year-old domestic shorthaired cat (**A**) and midthoracic kyphosis was seen in a 2-year-old English Bulldog (**B**). These animals had congenital vertebral lesions that caused a degree of vertebral segmental malalignment (arrows) that led to spinal canal stenosis with cord compression and resulting neurological signs. It is sometimes difficult to distinguish radiographically congenital/developmental lesions with or without secondary reactive bony changes from acute or chronic traumatic lesions. In many patients, minimal trauma causes an acute onset of clinical signs because of the acute spinal cord compressions.*

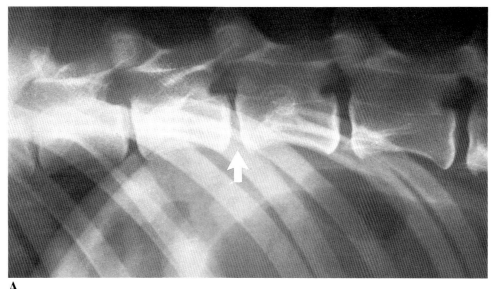

A

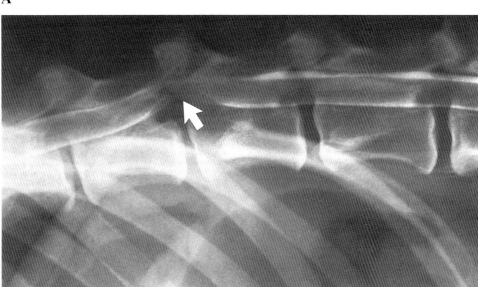

B

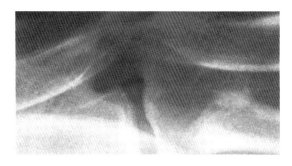

Figure 4-21.
Traumatic disc disease.
*A 5 year-old-German Shepherd Dog presented with an acute onset of hind limb paralysis thought to be due to trauma. The non-contrast radiographs showed some narrowing of the disc space at T12-13 (arrow) and a suggestion of bone density tissue in the dorsal portion of the disc space (**A**). The myelogram demonstrated the dorsal displacement of both the spinal cord and the subarachnoid columns (arrow) due to the traumatically herniated disc tissue (**B**). The calcified tissue within the disc space may be associated with a degenerated disc. However, this is more likely due to small avulsion fractures from the vertebral endplates as the annulus fibers have torn from the endplates.*

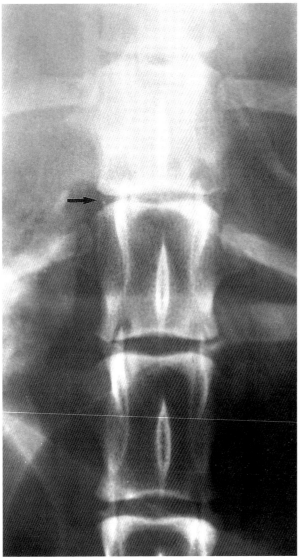

A

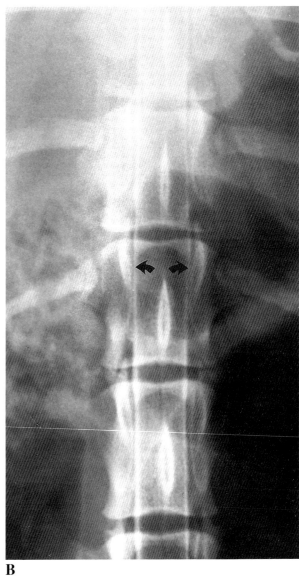

B

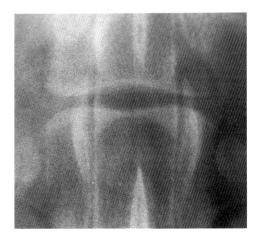

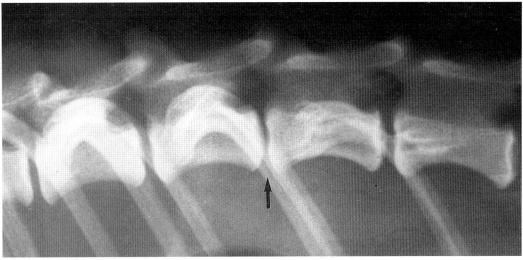

C

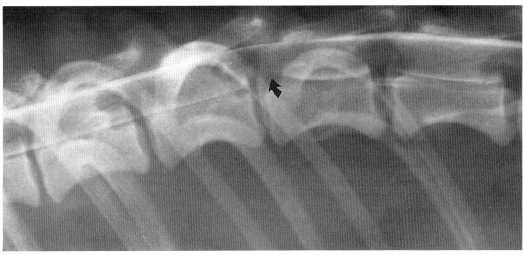

D

Figure 4-22.
Traumatic vertebral luxation.
*A mature mixed-breed dog was presented to the clinic with paralysis of the hind limbs. Non-contrast radiographs (**A**,**C**) showed only minimal disc space collapse at T12-13 (straight arrows). It is difficult to base a diagnosis on such a minimal radiographic change. Myelography was performed and the water-soluble contrast agent within the subarachnoid space demonstrated widening of the spinal cord on the ventrodorsal view (**B**, curved arrows) and elevation of the ventral contrast column and the spinal cord on the lateral view (**D**, curved arrow). While it was assumed, based on the history and the non-contrast radiographs, that there might be a traumatic luxation with possible disc protrusion at T12-13 , it is much safer to use myelography to determine the exact nature of the injury and the type of treatment required.*

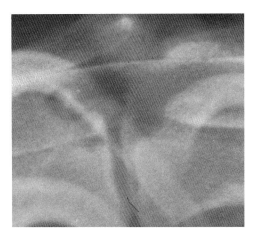

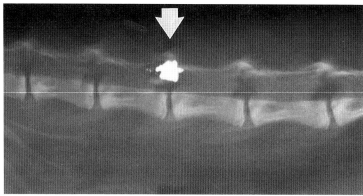

A

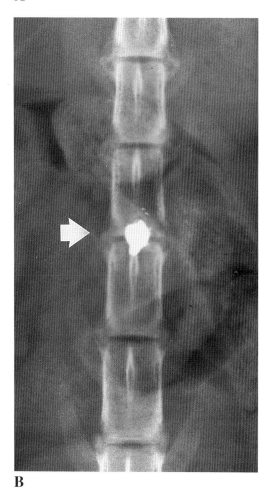

B

Figure 4-23.
Spinal gunshot injury.
Lateral **(A)** *and ventrodorsal* **(B)** *radiographs were made of a 10-month-old Siamese cat that was received in the clinic with a shoulder wound of unknown origin of 5 days duration. The clinical signs were those of a hind limb paralysis with exaggerated spinal reflexes and reduced response to pain sensation. The radiographs of the lumbar spine clearly showed the radiopaque foreign body (arrows). Examination of both orthogonal views is necessary to determine that the air-gun pellet lies within the spinal canal. The fractures of the dorsal laminae that permitted the pellet to enter the canal are difficult to identify.*

Figure 4-24.
Spinal gunshot injury.
Lateral (**A**) *and ventrodorsal* (**B**) *radiographs were made of an 8-year-old male Labrador Retriever that presented with a typical cauda equine syndrome after having been shot. The pathway made by the bullet was identified by the small metallic fragments within the soft tissues (arrows). The bullet passed through the sacral spinal canal. It is easy to imagine that a film artifact due to foreign material on the intensifying screens or gravel on the skin or in the feces of the animal could cause a similar pattern of radiodense shadows.*

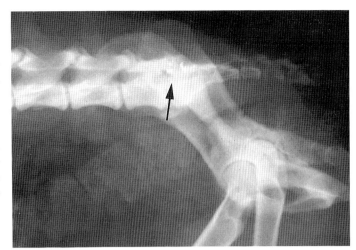

A

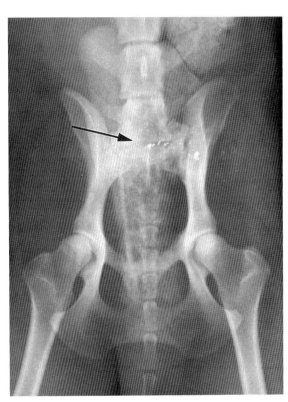

B

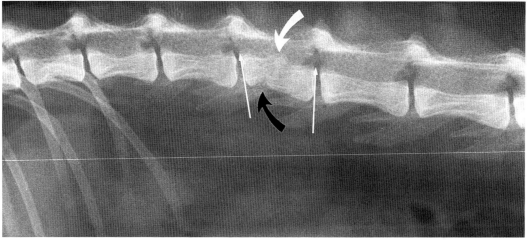

A

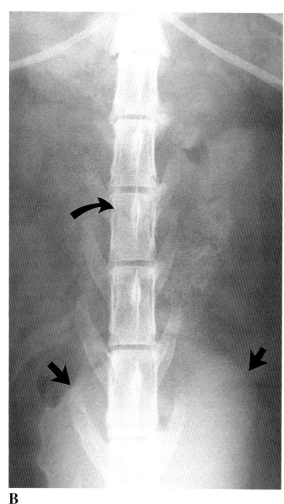

B

Figure 4-25.

Spinal pathologic fracture L3.

This mature spayed female domestic long-haired cat probably sustained minimal trauma, 2 weeks previously, based on an incomplete clinical history. At the time of presentation to the clinic, the cat had caudal paralysis with a lack of urinary bladder control. On the lateral radiograph (A), a partially compressed fracture involving the body of L3 was identified by a break in the ventral cortex, with inward folding (black curved arrow) and a more important bulging of bony tissue into the spinal canal (white curved arrow). The intervertebral discs are typically stronger than the bony vertebral segments and minimal trauma that causes a fracture within weakened vertebrae will leave the intervertebral disc spaces unaffected. Note that the vertebral endplates of the affected segments are no longer parallel to each other as a result of the compressive nature of the fracture (long white arrows). The fracture line is only partially visualized on the ventrodorsal view (B) because of the compressive nature of the lesion (black curved arrow). When a fracture causes bony tissue to be forced into the spinal canal there is cord compression with resulting transverse myelopathy, and neurological signs are noted in addition to pain from the fracture. The possibility of meningeal tearing or spinal cord trauma cannot be fully evaluated without the use of myelography. The urinary bladder is distended as part of the upper-motor neuron lesion in the pelvic area (B, black straight arrows).

Figure 4-26.
Intrapelvic hemorrhage.
*Radiographs of the pelvis of a 2-year-old domestic long-haired cat that had been missing for 2 days were made because palpation over the pelvic region proved to be very painful and the cat did not have a normal gait. On the ventrodorsal view (**A**), cranial displacement of the right hemipelvis was caused by luxation of the right sacroiliac joint (curved arrows) and separation of the symphysis pubis (curved arrows). The dislocations were not appreciated on the lateral view (**B**). However, on this view the most important clinical finding was the ventral displacement of the colon by an intrapelvic hematoma (large arrows).*

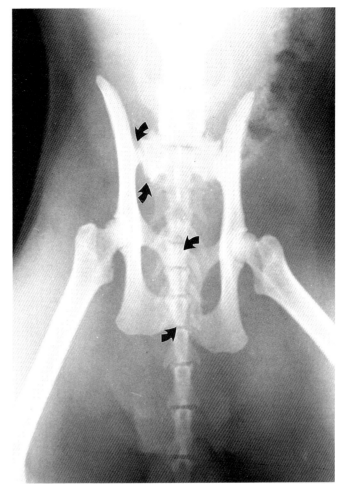

A

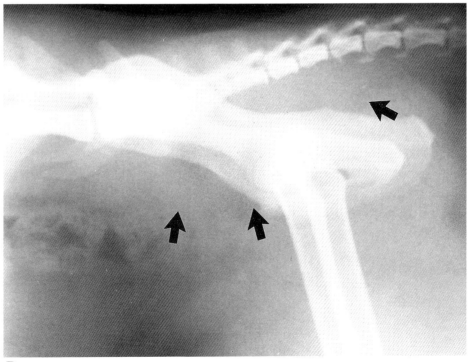

B

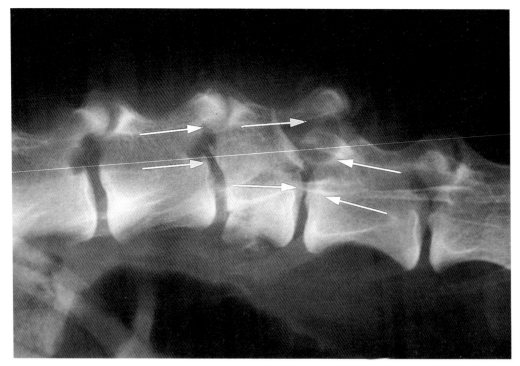

Figure 4-27.
Laminar vertebral fracture.
A 2-year-old Doberman Pinscher (Doberman) was hit by a car and presented at the clinic with no reflexes in the hind limbs and a cross extensor reflex in the forelimbs. A lateral radiograph of the spine showed a fracture of L4, with separation of the arch from the body. In fractures of this type the height of the spinal canal (long arrows) may be preserved, or may even become larger, offering some protection from injury to the spinal cord. Determination of spinal cord injury should be made from the results of the neurologic examination and not from the radiographic study.

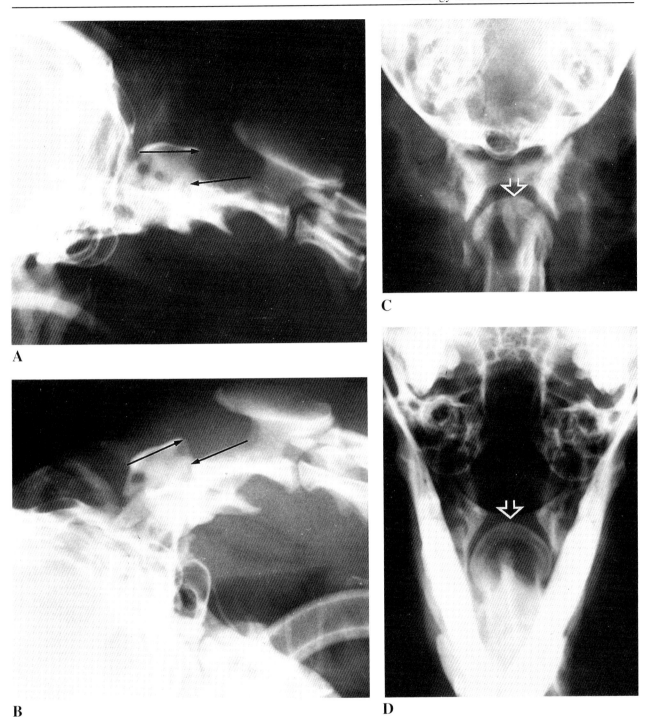

Figure 4-28.
Odontoid process lesion.
*This 1-year-old female Miniature Poodle sustained a rapid onset of tetraplegia following a fight with a larger dog. The lateral radiographs, made in a neutral (**A**) and hyperflexed position (**B**), clearly demonstrate the change in the height of the spinal canal but do not show the cause of the instability causing cord compression. The roof of the spinal canal in C1 and the dorsal surface of the odontoid process are marked (long black arrows). However, the ventrodorsal view of the cervical spine (**C**) and the "open-mouth" view (**D**) clearly show the absence of the odontoid process (hollow white arrows). The failure to identify the odontoid process on the radiograph is indicative of: (1) congenital aplasia, (2) presence of a cartilage model but with failure to ossify, or (3) fracture with displacement. These animals usually demonstrate clinical signs only following trauma that either exacerbates the congenital/developmental spinal instability or causes an odontoid fracture.*

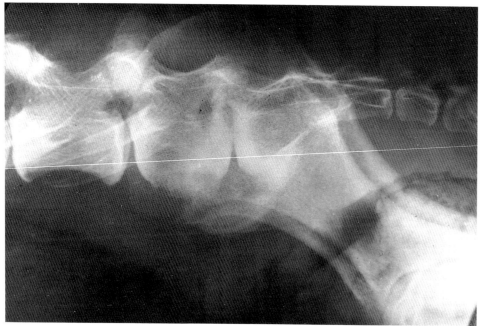

A

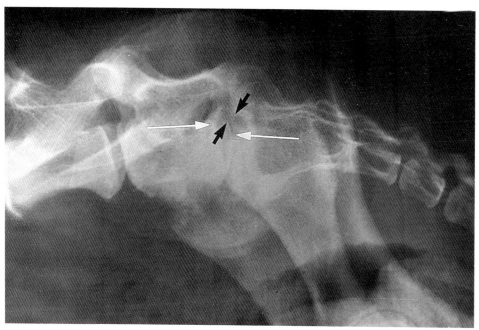

B

Figure 4-29.
Lumbosacral instability demonstrated with stress radiographs.
*A 3-year-old male German Shepherd Dog had a sudden onset of caudal paresis with suspicion of cauda equine syndrome. Stress radiographs made in a neutral position (**A**) and in hyperextended position (**B**) demonstrate dynamic instability at the lumbosacral junction (long white arrows) and narrowing of the spinal canal (short black arrows). This explains why these animals show pain when pressure is directed downward on the back.*

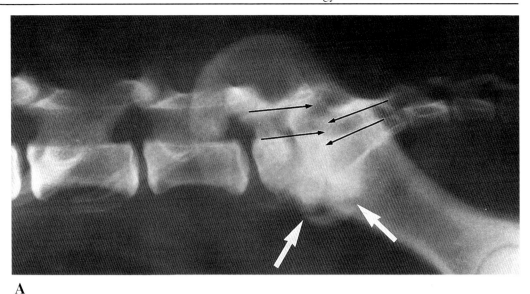

A

Figure 4-30.
Transitional sacral segment with instability.

Radiographs were made of the pelvic region of a 12-year-old male Schnauzer-cross that presented with back pain, nonweight-bearing on the left hind limb, decreased conscious proprioceptive sensation of the left hind limb, and constipation. The owner was uncertain how long the dog had these signs and did not know if the onset of the signs had been sudden. Malalignment of the sacral segments was indicated by the disruption of the floor of the spinal canal (black arrows). Diagnosis was complicated because of the presence of reactive vertebral spondylosis ventral to the sacrum at what appeared to be a junction between the first and second sacral segments (white arrows). Differential diagnosis included: (1) chronic fracture of the sacrum with malalignment of the fragments and healing callus, (2) congenital transitional sacral segments with heavy reactive spondylosis due to degenerating disc with secondary slippage of the caudal segment, (3) congenital transitional sacral segments that formed with segmental instability and malalignment, and (4) fracture following congenital, developmental, or degenerative L-S disc disease with callus formation.

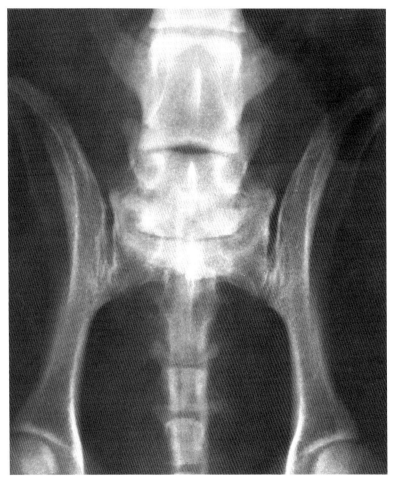

B

Even in the absence of an exact etiology in this dog, important clinical information — malalignment of the sacral segments with resulting stenosis of the sacral spinal canal (black arrows) — is available on the radiographs. Stress views could indicate whether there is dynamic instability with accentuated canal stenosis associated with the disease. This is important information because it suggests whether treatment is to be limited to decompression or whether surgical stabilization is required as well. This dog was thought to have a congenital transitional lumbosacral vertebral segment with secondary instability.

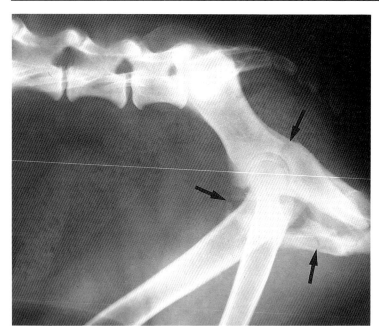

A

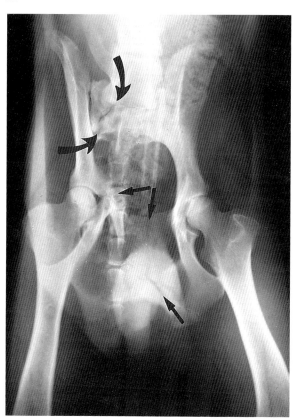

B

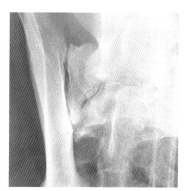

Figure 4-31.
Sacral fracture.
*Pelvic radiographs were made of a 3-year-old male mix-breed who returned home ataxic in the pelvic limbs, after being missing for 7 days. Crepitus was detected on pelvic examination. The pubic, ischial, and right acetabular fractures (straight arrows) are best seen on the lateral view (**A**). The more important lesion is the fracture of the sacrum (curved arrows) visible on the ventro-dorsal view (**B**). This lesion caused the cauda equina syndrome.*

Figure 4-32.
Rib fractures.
A 7-year-old Beagle was presented with a history of trauma, 1 week earlier. Thoracic radiographs showed the typical appearance of disruption of the rib shadows with fractures (arrows). The fractures are bilateral and present the typical radiographic appearance that is often an incidental finding following thoracic trauma. Despite the severity and number of ribs fractured, they usually heal without treatment or difficulty.

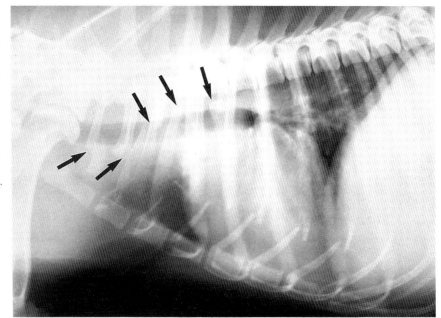

A

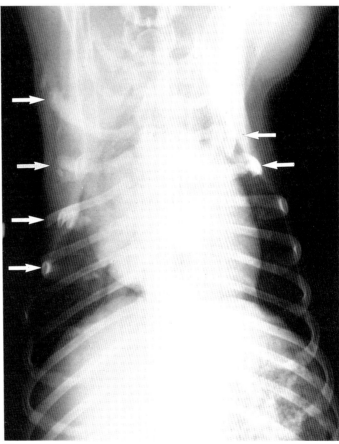

B

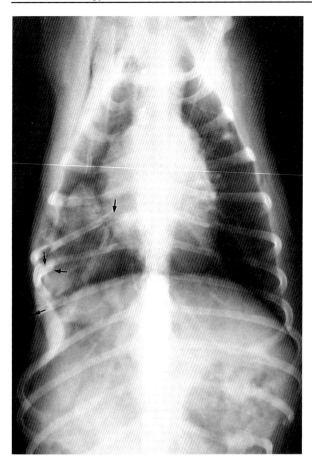

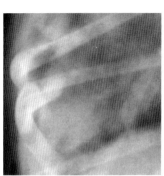

Figure 4-33.
Rib fractures.
This is a dorsoventral radiograph of the thorax of a 3-year-old female Sheltie that was bitten by a larger dog. She received trauma to the right rib cage with resulting broken ribs, pulmonary contusion, minimal pneumothorax, and subcutaneous emphysema as evident on the radiograph. The rib fractures are characterized by differences in width of intercostal spaces and disruption of rib shadows (arrows). The dog recovered with medical care.

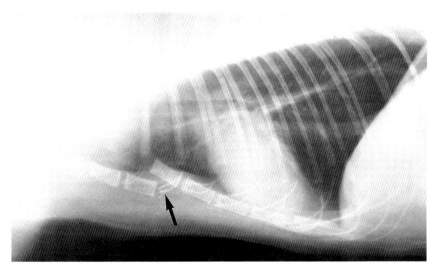

Figure 4-34.
Sternal luxation.
A 6-year-old male domestic short-haired cat was radiographed because of suspected dyspnea. The luxation between the sternal segments (arrow) was an incidental finding but was thought to be associated with recent thoracic trauma because of the absence of any reactive changes associated with the injury. Sternal trauma usually causes only minimal clinical signs.

Figure 4-35.
Sternal congenital anomaly.
*Clinically, palpation revealed an abnormal rib cage in this 3-month-old male Himalayan kitten with normal heart sounds. The kitten was thought to have been attacked by a dog in the household. Radiographic examination of the thorax showed a severe deformity of the thoracic cage. As a result, the heart shadow had shifted markedly to the left (**A**, black arrows) and dorsally (**B**, white arrows). This congenital abnormality of the sternum and rib cage is called pectus excavatum and is often associated with abnormal diaphragmatic attachment. Pericardial-diaphragmatic hernia may be found in patients with severe sternal anomalies.*

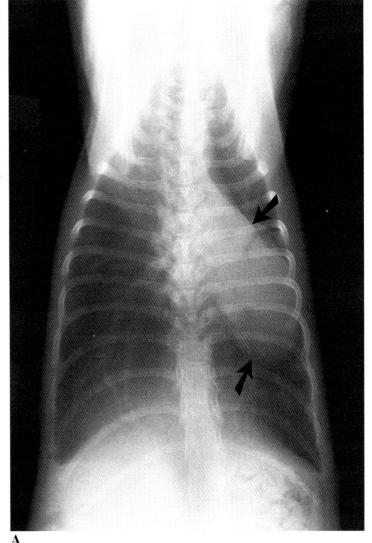

A

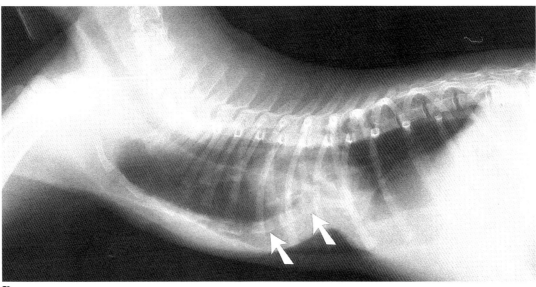

B

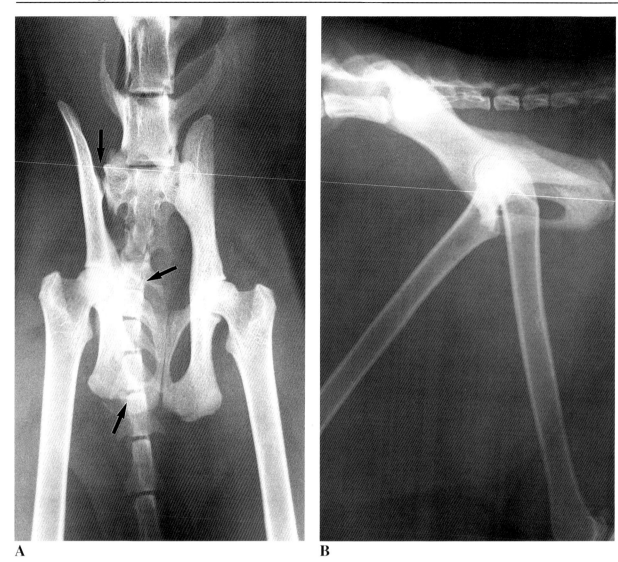

A   B

Figure 4-36.
Pelvic fracture-luxations.
*A cat with hindleg lameness was brought into the clinic by someone other than the owner. Radiographs were made of the pelvis, and a frequent pattern of trauma was noted. A sacroiliac luxation (arrow) and pubic and ischial fractures (arrows) were noted, all on the right side (**A**). The right hemipelvis was freed by the trauma and displaced cranially by muscle pull. Note that both hip joints are unaffected by the trauma. The bladder is only faintly seen on the lateral radiograph (**B**). Possible injury to that organ should always be evaluated in a patient with pelvic trauma.*

Figure 4-37.
Pelvic fracture-luxations.
A ventrodorsal radiograph was made of the pelvis of a 1-year-old male Shepherd-cross that was hit by a car, 3 days earlier. The dog was unable to support weight on the rear limbs when presented at the clinic. The pelvis was divided by a luxation of the right sacroiliac joint (arrow) and an important fracture through the left acetabulum (arrow) with resulting cranial displacement at the right side. Anatomical reduction of the acetabular fracture is important in preventing secondary post-traumatic arthrosis.

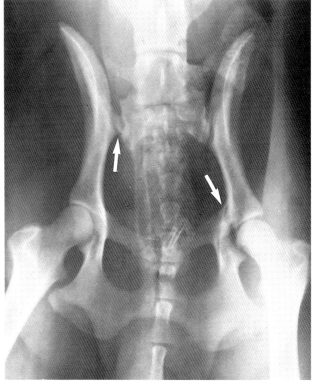

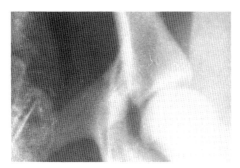

Figure 4-38.
Acetabular fractures.
A ventrodorsal radiograph of the pelvis of a 1-year-old female Saint Bernard was made following collision with a car. Fracture lines were seen to involve multiple bones, including, most importantly, both acetabulae (arrows). Note the partial luxation of the femoral heads, probably indicating pre-existing coxo-femoral instability due to hip dysplasia.

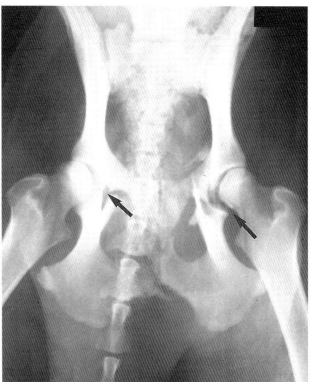

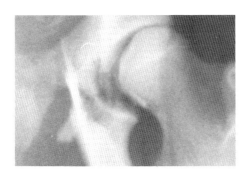

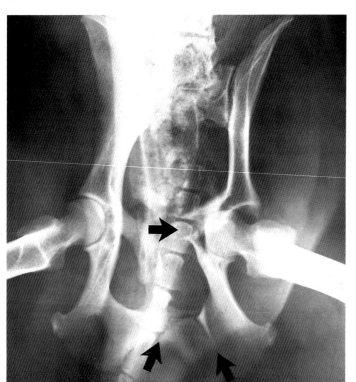

A

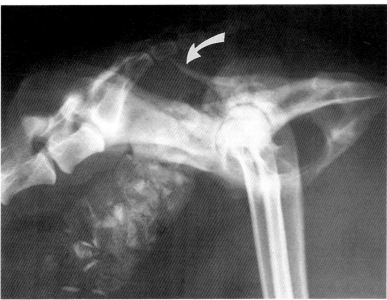

B

Figure 4-39.
Acetabular fracture.
*Ventrodorsal (**A**) and lateral (**B**) radiographs of the pelvis of a young mix-breed dog were made following pelvic trauma. The left femoral head is displaced medially through the fractured acetabulum (A, black arrow) causing narrowing of the pelvic canal. Additional fractures involve the left ischium (A, black arrows). The lateral radiograph shows a fragment of iliac bone displaced dorsally (B, white arrow). The time of injury was not known. The presence of dense fecal material within the colon probably results from obstipation because of painful defecation and suggests an injury of some days duration. Malpositioning of the ventrodorsal view is common in examinations of patients with pelvic fractures. It is often helpful to place the pelvic limbs into a flexed position since this may be less painful.*

Figure 4-40.
Ischial fracture.
A 9-month-old male mixed-breed was painful in the left rear limb. The single fracture of the left ischium (arrows) partially involves the growth plates for these apophyseal growth centers. Note that the fracture lines do not appear to involve the left acetabulum. Single fractures are more common in skeletally immature animals in which the bones still have a degree of mobility prior to fracturing. A lead shield was used for gonadal protection during the radiographic examination.

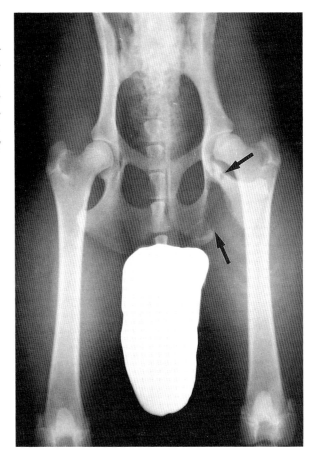

Figure 4-41.
Capital physeal and greater trochanteric fractures.
A 6-month-old male kitten was hit by a car and refused to use the left hind limb. A ventrodorsal radiograph of the pelvis demonstrated a slipped capital epiphysis (straight arrows) plus avulsion of the greater trochanter (curved arrows). Examination of all of the growth centers of the pelvis and proximal femur is important in trauma patients.

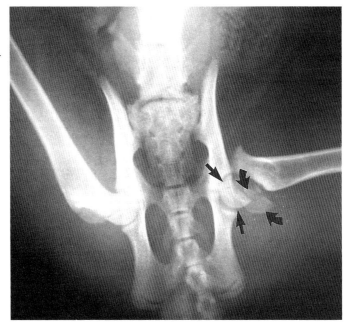

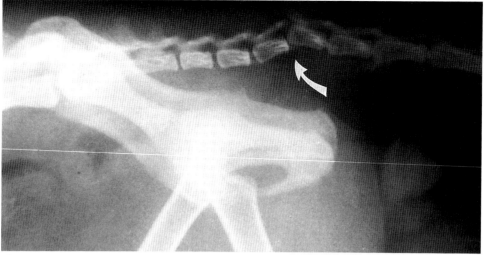

A

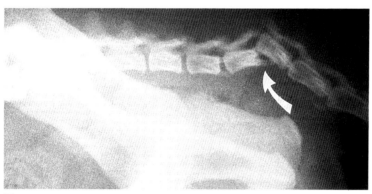

B

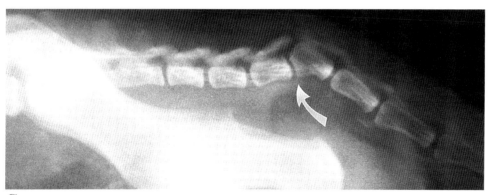

C

Figure 4-42.
Caudal segment fracture-luxation.
*This 1-year-old, castrated male domestic short-haired cat had not walked normally for several weeks and was finally presented for examination. Palpation of the tail was thought to be abnormal and radiographs were made. A fracture-luxation (curved arrows) at Cg 3-4 was seen (**A**). The lesion was reradiographed 2 weeks later (**B**). Stabilization of the fracture/luxation occurred 2 months later (**C**). This is an example of how a traumatically induced malformed vertebral segment when identified without a clinical history of trauma, might be misdiagnosed as a congenital anomaly. The injury was caudal in location and apparently without severe soft tissue damage since it resulted only in a flaccid tail.*

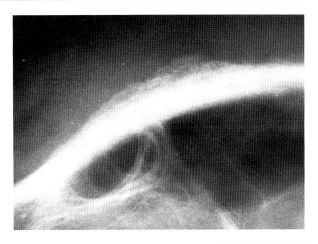

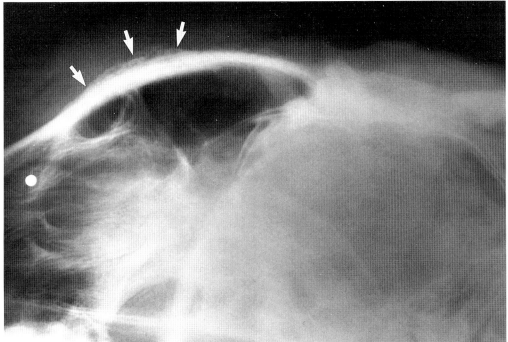

Figure 4-43.
Post-traumatic osteomyelitis.
A 5-year-old male short-haired German Pointer was injured in the head and subsequently developed a draining lesion in the temporal region. Drainage was controlled with antibiotic therapy, but reoccurred when this therapy was stopped. Radiographs of the head were made. The lateral view demonstrated soft tissue swelling over the right frontal bone with a mixed productive and destructive frontal bone lesion (arrows). The thickened frontal bone with laminar-type periosteal reactive bone formation is supportive of the clinical diagnosis of osteomyelitis. The shotgun pellets were probably not related to the bone infection.

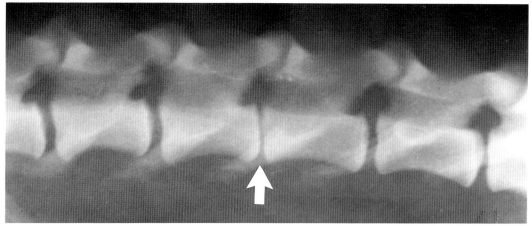

A

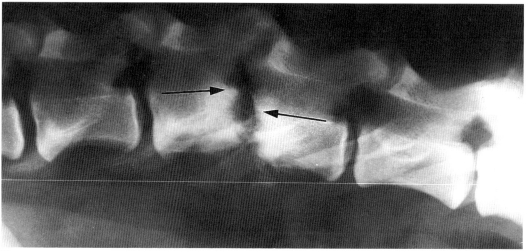

B

Figure 4-44.
Traumatic vertebral luxation with secondary discospondylitis.

A 4-year-old male Golden Retriever was radiographed after being struck by a car. Marked collapse of the L3-4 disc space was noted (A, white arrow), without evidence of segmental malalignment or any bony fragmentation suggesting traumatic luxation. It was reported that the dog could not move the pelvic limbs. The dog was treated with corticosteroids. When the dog was presented 4 weeks later, it was ambulatory on the thoracic limbs only, showed marked muscle wasting, had decreased proprioception in the pelvic limbs, increased patellar tendon reflexes in the pelvic limbs, and positive pain perception in the pelvic limbs. Radiographic examination was repeated (B). The radiographic image had changed dramatically, with marked widening of the affected disc space, destruction of the vertebral endplates, and malalignment of the vertebral segments (black arrows). This is an example of a traumatic injury with subsequent development of inflammatory disc disease. Cultures of urine, blood, and material obtained from the disc space under fluoroscopic control, all grew Staphylococcus aureus *that was penicillin-sensitive. There was an increase in number of white blood cells.*

It is common for hematogenous osteomyelitis (discospondylitis) to occur at sites of trauma or disc degeneration. It is assumed that a secondary capillary bed that has grown into the disc space is not normal and provides locations for emboli to colonize. In this dog, this could be the explanation for the infectious lesion secondary to the trauma. The dog was prescribed 1 gram oxacillin TID and remained on that dosage for over 1 month. It was eventually necessary to perform a hemilaminectomy, to curette the affected disc space, and to install a double 4-pin KE device for vertebral stabilization. Postoperatively, the patient was without neurological improvement, and became a major nursing problem during the phase of healing.

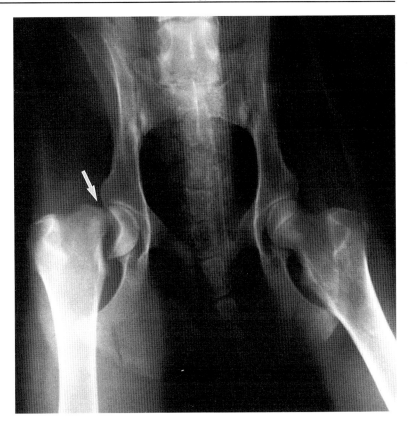

Figure 4-45.
Capital femoral physeal fracture.
A ventrodorsal pelvic radiograph of a 9-month-old male Doberman Pinscher (Doberman) that was hit by a truck revealed a Type-I physeal fracture of the right proximal femur (arrow). The head of the femur remained within the acetabulum. These physeal fractures are particularly difficult to treat successfully because of the loss of blood supply to the capital epiphysis due to the location of the physeal plate within the torn joint capsule.

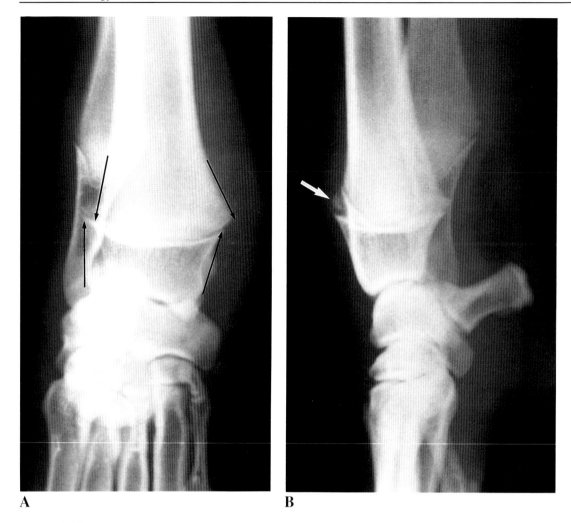

A   **B**

Figure 4-46.

Distal radial physeal fracture.

*Radiographs of the distal forelimb of a 6-month-old puppy showed a Type-I physeal fracture of the distal radius, with resulting minimal fragment malposition (**A**, black arrows). The soft tissue swelling is of assistance in locating the bony injury. It is not possible to determine from the radiograph the maximum degree of displacement of the physis and thus the extent of the injury to the soft tissues. At the time of radiography, the displacement between the epiphysis and metaphysis had been reduced resulting in an almost anatomical position. Note the small bony fragment on the cranial surface of the distal radial metaphysis (**B**, white arrow) that is important in determining the site of the trauma.*

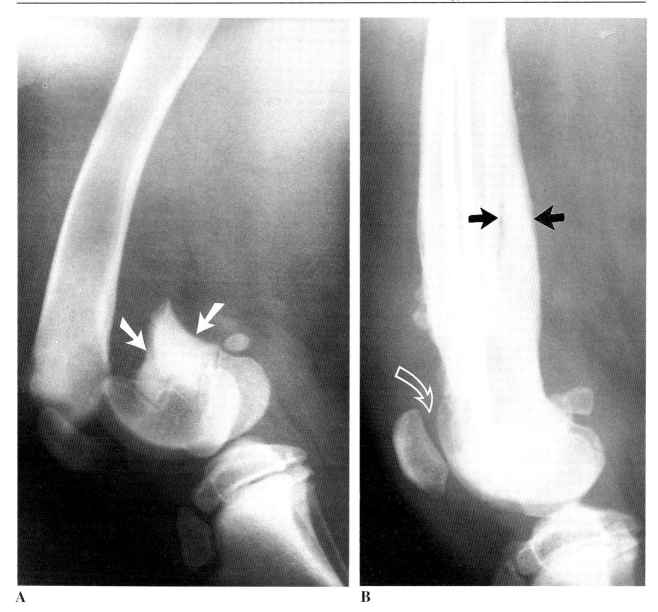

A   B

Figure 4-47.
Distal femoral physeal fracture.
*Radiographs of the distal femur in a 3-month-old mixed-breed dog showed a Type-II physeal fracture (**A**). This type of physeal fracture is characterized by a triangular shaped metaphyseal fragment (solid white arrows) that remains attached to the distal femoral epiphysis. The second study was made 4 weeks post-stabilization and showed an increase in bone density that is primarily due to the newly formed callus (**B**). The periosteum in young puppies is loosely attached to the cortex and strips easily with an injury of this type. The thickness of the massive callus proximal to the fracture site is determined by the location of the original cortex and the torn periosteum (black arrows). Note that in healing, the physeal plate has closed. The affected femur will be shortened in length, but the dog will compensate through greater extension of the stifle joint while walking. The femoro-patellar joint (B, hollow white arrow) is not as closely fitting as it should be, and may require additional surgical therapy in the future to prevent development of a post-traumatic arthrosis.*

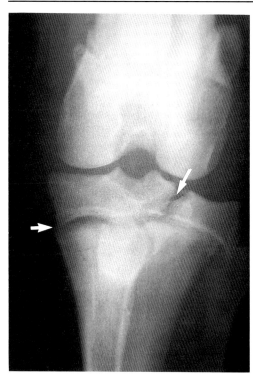

Figure 4-48.
Proximal tibial physeal fracture.
A 9-month-old male Irish Wolfhound was hit by a car and presented with a swollen left hind limb. A caudocranial radiograph of the stifle joint demonstrated a Type-III physeal fracture of the proximal tibia, with the fracture line passing through the medial portion of the physeal plate (arrow) and exiting into the joint (arrow). In addition to physeal character of this fracture, this is also an intra-articular fracture.

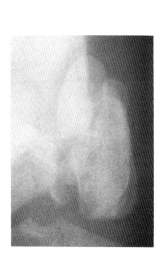
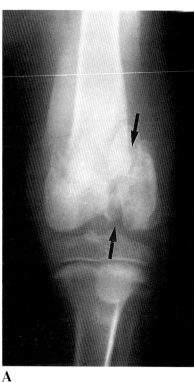
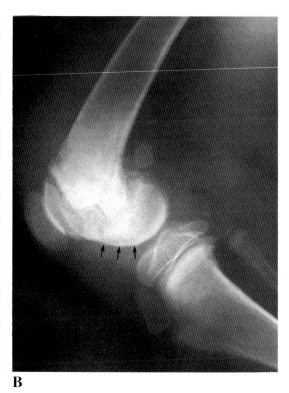

A   **B**

Figure 4-49.
Distal femoral physeal fracture.
*Injury involving the distal femoral growth centers in a 3-month-old female Doberman Pinscher (Doberman) puppy was radiographically diagnosed. The fracture line extended vertically through the metaphysis, physis, and epiphyses (large arrows) and separated the lateral condyle (**A**). In addition, both femoral condyles were rotated caudally, as seen on the lateral view (arrows) suggesting that there is complete physeal separation as well (**B**). The fracture is, therefore, a combination of a Type-I and a Type-IV growth plate injury. These injuries do not have the same serious consequences as the growth plate injuries in the distal radius and ulna where the paired bones must both grow to a similar length.*

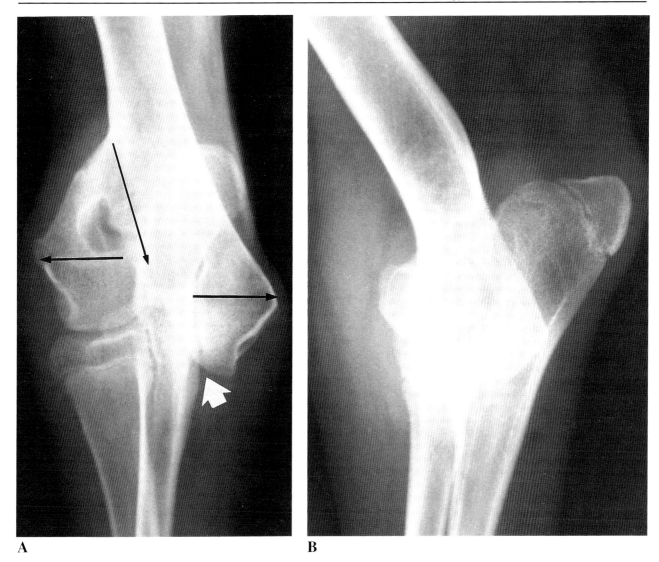

A   B

Figure 4-50.
Healed distal humeral physeal fracture with malunion.
A 5-month-old Dalmation puppy had a chronically sore elbow joint because of a healed malunion Type-IV physeal fracture of the distal humerus. Dislocation of the lateral humeral condyle proximally has resulted in a marked displacement of the growth plate in the distal humerus (A, horizontal black arrows). The healed fracture line is marked (A, vertical black arrow). The resulting subluxation of the trochlear notch of the ulna (B) is due to the malarticulation and displacement of the medial humeral condyle distally (A, white arrow). The malarticulation led to development of a severe post-traumatic arthrosis. Note the soft tissue swelling due to capsular thickening.

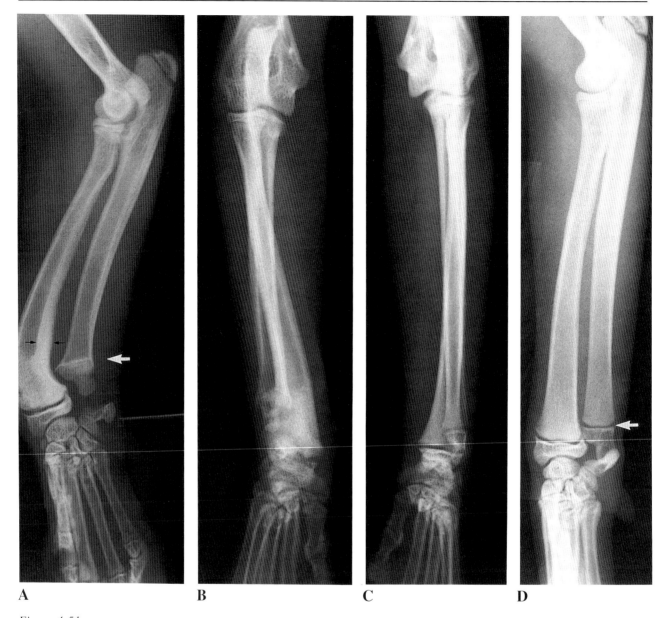

A   B   C   D

Figure 4-51.
Post-traumatic distal ulnar growth abnormality.
*Radiographs were made of the clinically abnormal forelimb of a lame 4-month-old female kitten in which there was no history of injury (**A, B**). Clinically, the right forepaw was deviated laterally (externally) while the leg appeared to be bowed. Comparison with the contralateral normal forelimb (**C, D**)was helpful in reaching a diagnosis. Premature closure of the distal ulnar growth plate had resulted in marked shortening of the ulna.*
This is characterized by: (1) proximal displacement of the styloid process of the ulna, (2) closure of the distal ulnar physis (white arrow), (3) curvature of the radius with thickening of the medial and caudal cortex (black arrows) due to abnormal stress lines and piëzo-electric effect, and (4) early radiocarpal luxation. Notice the external rotation of the affected forelimb as seen on the craniocaudal view (B). The elbow joint remained unaffected in this cat. Lesions of this type are more common in dogs, but are seen in cats as well. Surgical treatment consists of ulnar osteotomy to permit separation of the ulnar fragments and artificial lengthening of that bone. At a later time, a radial wedge osteotomy is necessary to correct the bowing of the radius. Regardless of the success in treatment of this limb angulation, the injury to the articular surfaces of the radiocarpal joint has already occurred, and a degree of secondary joint disease will develop.

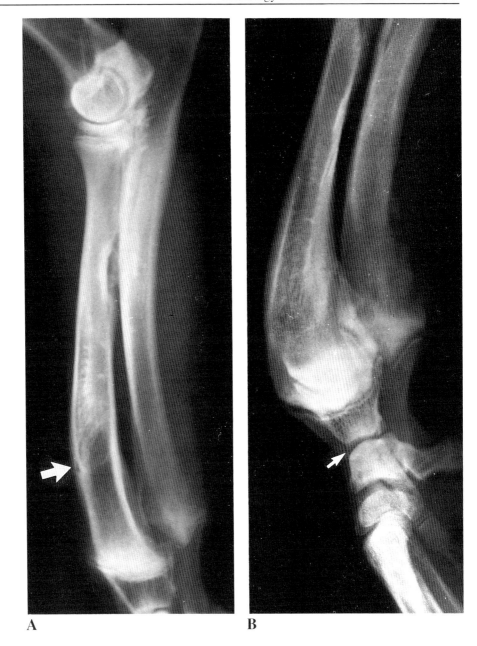

A   B

Figure 4-52.
Post-traumatic distal ulnar growth abnormality.
*Lateral radiographs were made of the distal forelimb of a Shepherd mix-breed dog that received an injury to the forelimb at 9 weeks of age. The radiographs were made at 5 months of age (**A**) and at 8 months of age (**B**). The earlier radiograph shows healing of a mid-shaft radial fracture (arrow) and beginning overgrowth of the radius. The second study clearly shows the continued overgrowth of the radius. Note that the ulnar growth plate is still open. The problem is not a complete closure of the distal ulnar growth plate, but rather an injury resulting in the unequal growth between the two bones. The articular surface of the distal radial epiphysis is seen to maintain contact with the articular surface of the radial carpal bone in a near-normal manner; however, this is a site for potential joint disease in the future (small arrow). This patient is a good example of the change in the thickness of the radial cortices as the lines of force change with the bowing of the bone. As more weight is borne on the caudal cortex, it becomes thicker.*

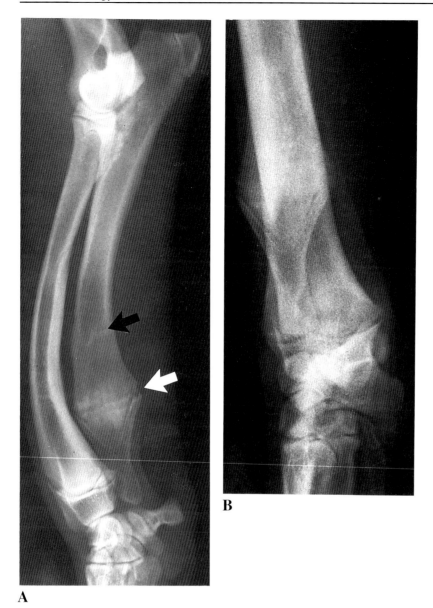

A

B

Figure 4-53.

Post-traumatic distal ulnar growth abnormality.

*A 7-month-old female Labrador Retriever was presented with an obvious cur-
vature and marked external rotation of the right forelimb (**A, B**). The left forelimb was clinically normal by comparison (**C, D**). Lateral radiographs should
include both the carpal and elbow joints to evaluate possible secondary injury
to either joint. The unnoticed traumatic injury to the forelimb had resulted in
injury to the distal ulna and the dense scar in the ulnar diaphysis (black arrow)
suggested a healed fracture. The distal ulnar physis was still open (white
arrow), but the metaphysis was not fully mineralized. The resulting deformity
resembles a "retained cartilage core" in the distal ulna and suggests delayed
growth due to a similar cause.*

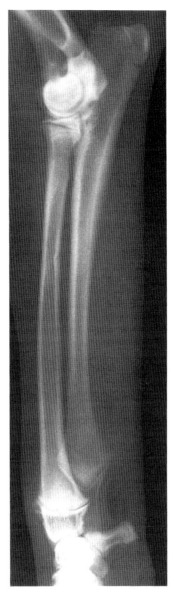

C

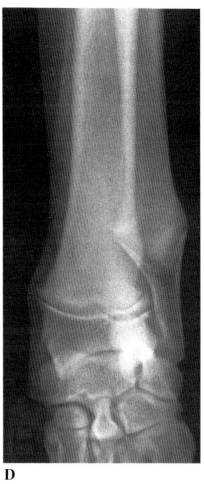

D

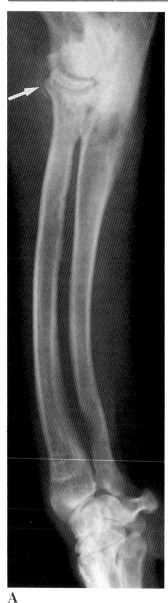
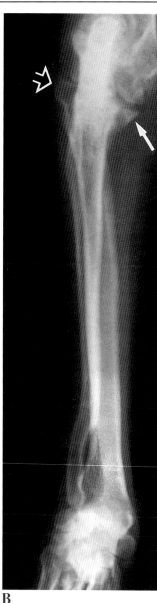

Figure 4-54.
Post-traumatic distal ulnar growth abnormality.
*The right forelimb (**A, B**) of this 5-month-old German Shepherd Dog was shorter than the left and there was marked outward rotation of the foot, with cranial bowing of the antebrachium. These physical findings are typical of those resulting from a shortened ulna secondary to early closure of the distal growth plate. For reasons of comparison, radiographs of the normal left forelimb were also made (**C, D**). Early closure of the distal ulnar and radial growth plates was obvious when compared with the "open" growth plates in the normal limb. In this patient, examination of the elbow joint proved to be important because the radial head of the affected leg had attempted to luxate laterally (hollow arrow) with consequent remodeling of the proximal radius and ulna (solid arrows) and development of secondary joint disease. As a result of this elbow deformity reducing the stress in the affected forelimb, development of the injury in the distal portion of the limb was only minimal. The site of the original injury is not clearly suggested by these radiographs, but there is an apparent disruption of the proximal ulnar cortex that suggests a healing fracture. If that were the case, a proximal injury in the limb caused closure of the growth plate distally. This is thought to happen frequently.*

A

B

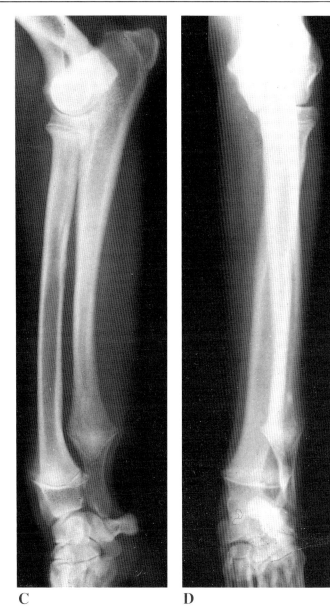

C

D

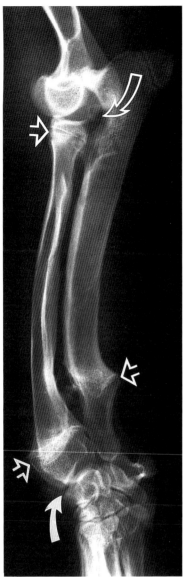

A

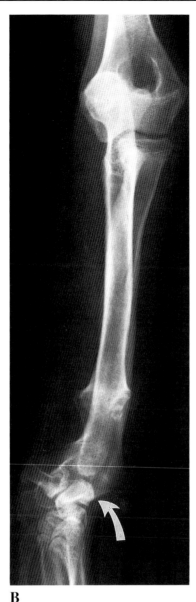

B

Figure 4-55.

Post-traumatic forelimb growth abnormality.
*A 3-month-old male Australian Shepherd Dog fractured the distal radius and ulna in the left forelimb at 6 weeks of age. The leg was placed in a cast from 3 weeks until 12 weeks after the accident. When the cast was removed, lateral deviation of the forelimb was noted. Radiographs were made of the affected limb (**A, B**) and the clinically normal right limb for comparison (**C, D**). Severe architectural abnormalities were noted in the affected limb secondary to apparent early closure of the growth plates in the distal radius and ulna, and in the proximal radius (hollow straight arrows). Proximal displacement of the ulnar styloid process has caused the distal radial articular surface to slip away cranially, resulting in malalignment with the proximal row of carpal bones (curved solid arrows). The foot has achieved an external rotation of almost 90 degrees. The radial head has displaced the humeral condyles away from the trochlear notch of the ulna (curved hollow arrow), with subsequent subluxation of the elbow. This animal is an example of how secondary growth deformity is dependent on (1) which growth plates are injured, (2) the age of the patient at the time of injury, and (3) the level and nature of injury.*

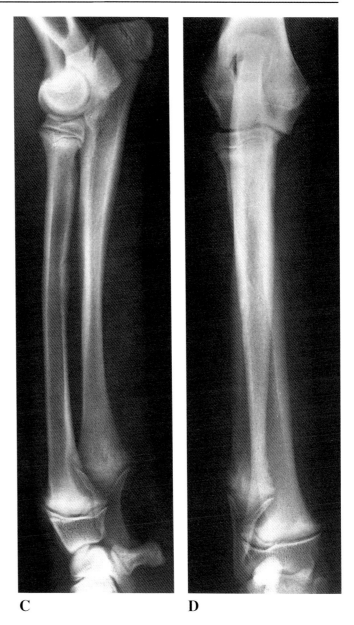

C   D

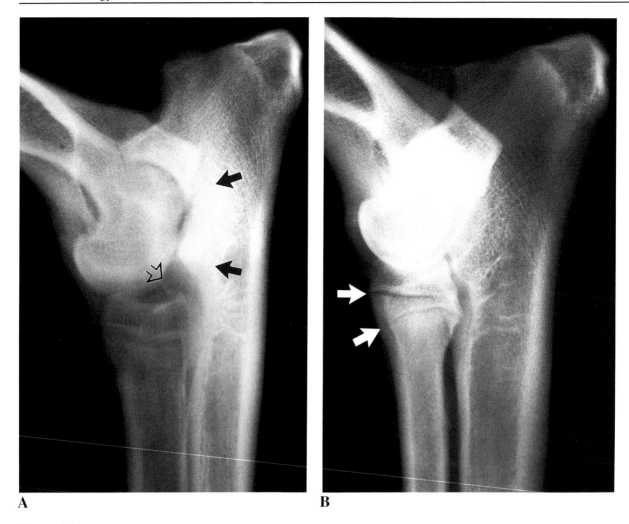

A   B

Figure 4-56.
Post-traumatic proximal radial growth plate abnormality.
*Delayed growth in the proximal radial growth plate in a 7-month-old female Irish Wolfhound resulted in shortening of the radius in the affected limb (**A**). In the normal limb (**B**), the growth plate of the proximal radius was still open (white arrows). The shortened radius has displaced the humeral condyles distally due to ligamentous attachments and the force of the condyles has destroyed the medial coronoid process of the normally growing ulna (open arrow). Radiographic signs of secondary joint are visible, with marked sclerosis in the proximal ulna adjacent to the trochlear notch (black arrows).*

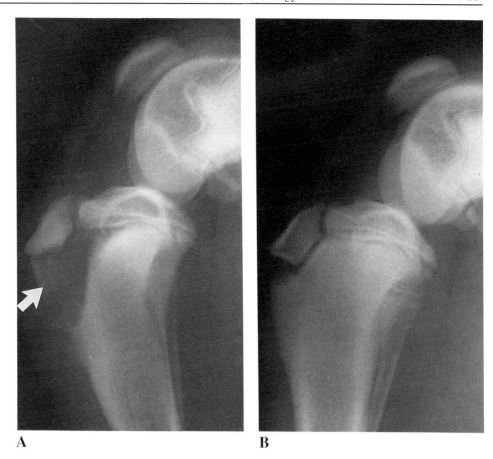

A   **B**

Figure 4-57.
Tibial crest avulsion fracture.
*A 5-month-old male Rhodesian Ridgeback was noted to be lame in the left rear limb. Lateral radiographs of both stifle joints showed an avulsion of the tibial crest (arrow) in the affected limb (**A**), and a normal-appearing apophyseal growth center in the normal limb (**B**). The injury was acute and fragmented calcified cartilage from the growth plate is seen between the fragment and the host bone. When displacement is minimal, it is important to make a radiograph of the normal limb for comparison to more accurately evaluate suspected injury to the growth centers of the limb.*

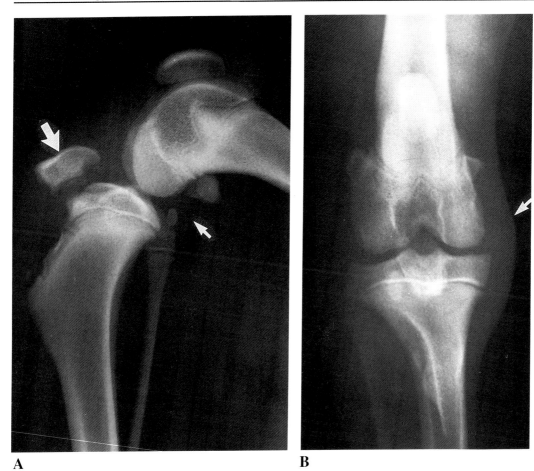

A   **B**

Figure 4-58.
Avulsion fracture tibial crest.
An 8-month-old male mix-breed dog was examined with lameness of the right hind limb. The joint capsule of the stifle was thickened and palpation proved to be painful. Radiographs of the stifle joint (A, B) clearly demonstrated an avulsion fracture of the tibial crest (large arrow), with resulting proximal patellar displacement. No evidence of instability of the joint was noted, although joint capsule swelling was evident (small arrows). The physeal growth plates were still open. The fracture bed is smooth suggesting that the injury is chronic and, as a result, replacement of the tibial crest may be more difficult than would appear from the radiographic study.

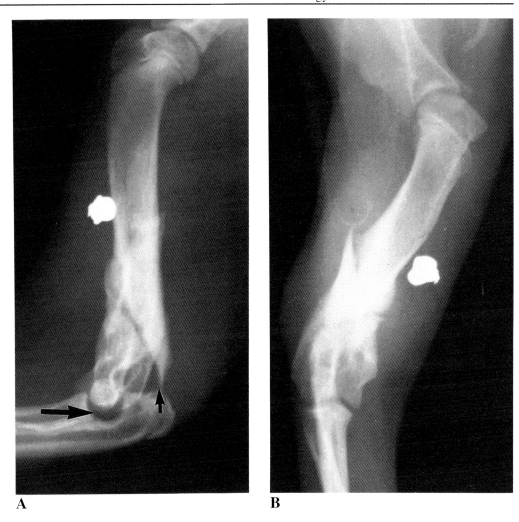

A   B

Figure 4-59.
Healing humeral gunshot fracture.
Radiographs of the forelimb of this young cat demonstrated a healing oblique mid-shaft humeral fracture, with over-riding of the fracture fragments (short arrow). The metallic bullet had remained in the soft tissues adjacent to the fracture. It looked like a soft pellet fired from an air-gun. The apparent subluxation of the elbow joint (long arrow) may relate to muscle atrophy and stress from the positioning for the radiographic study. However, it cannot be excluded that this abnormality is also a result of the earlier traumatic incident, and, therefore, should be further evaluated.

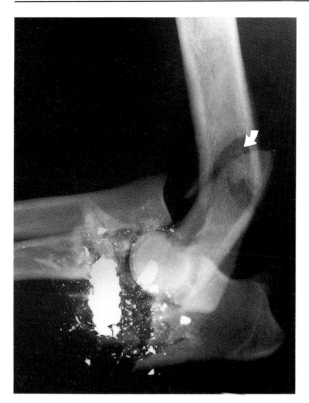

Figure 4-60.
Elbow fracture-luxation due to gunshot.
A lateral radiograph of the elbow joint of a male Malamute-cross was made when the dog returned home lame, having been missing from home for two weeks. The comminuted ulnar fracture and luxation of the radial head are easily seen. The pattern of this injury and the distribution of the particles of the bullet identify this gunshot injury as being from a high-velocity missile. The fracture of the distal humerus (arrow) supports the concept that, because of the nature of this high velocity injury, bones at a distance from the bullet tract may be fractured without having been struck directly by the missile.

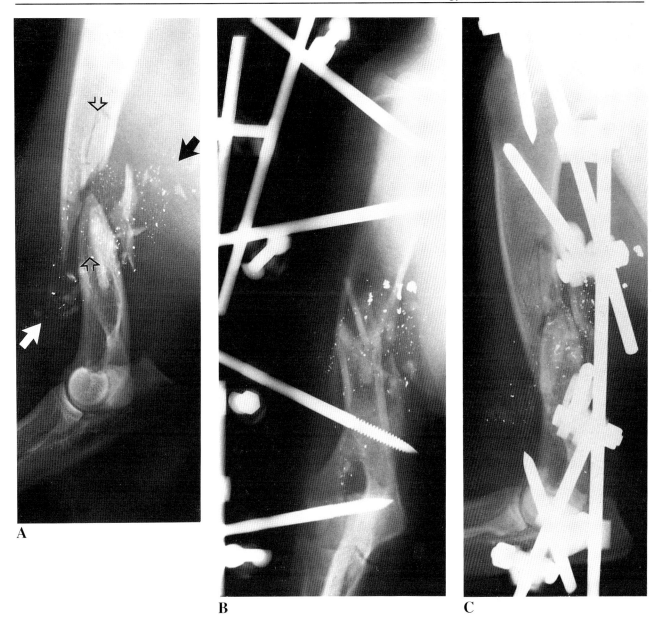

Figure 4-61.
Humeral gunshot fracture.
*A lateral radiograph of the forelimb of a mature dog with an open fracture of the mid-diaphysis of the humerus (**A**) reveals severe comminution of the fracture (hollow arrows) and the pathway of metallic fragments from the high velocity bullet (solid arrows). The post-stabilization radiographs demonstrate the use of a full Kirschner apparatus (**B**, **C**), with two threaded pins in the distal fragment and two threaded pins in the proximal fragment. Slight medial and cranial angulation of the major distal fragment is present.*

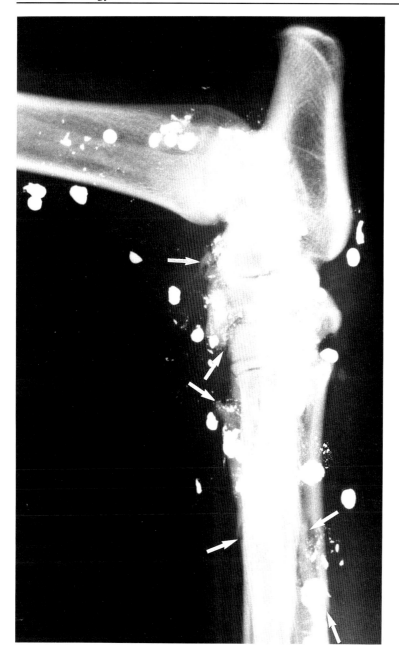

Figure 4-62.
Tarsal shotgun injury.
A lateral radiograph of the tarsal region of a hunting dog shows the effect of being struck by a large number of low-velocity missiles from a shotgun. Usually massive injury to the soft tissues results, with lesser injury to the bones. In addition, multiple comminuted fractures are seen (arrows) due to the close range of the gun at firing.

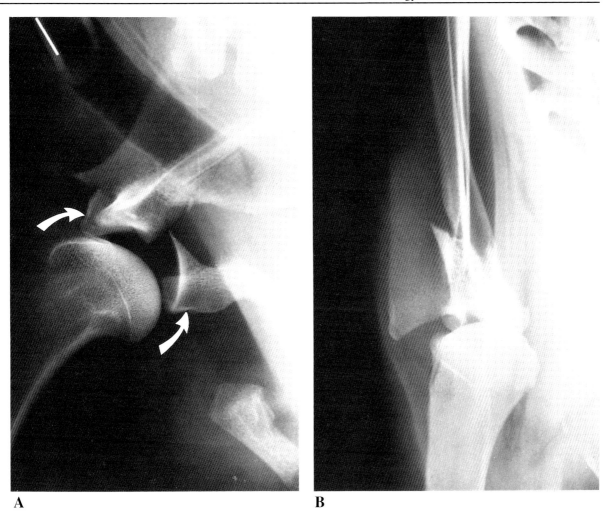

A   **B**

Figure 4-63.
Scapular fracture.
A 1-year-old Doberman Pinscher (Doberman) was hit by a car 4 days earlier and was presented to the clinic unable to bear weight on the right forelimb. A comminuted articular fracture of the distal scapula with caudal and lateral displacement of the two major distal fracture segments was noted (arrows). The destruction of the glenoid cavity is extensive.

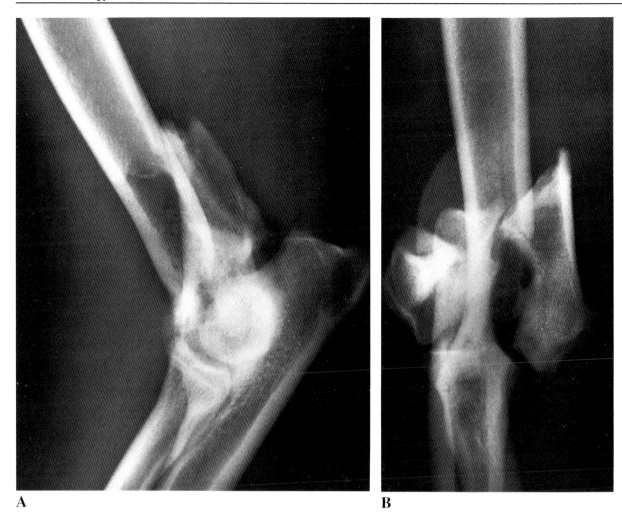

A   **B**

Figure 4-64.
Distal humeral fracture.
*A 1-year-old Brittany (Brittany Spaniel) jumped from a height of over 2 meters and presented with severe pain and swelling of the elbow joint. Crepitation was obvious. Lateral (**A**) and craniocaudal (**B**) radiographs showed the "Y" type fracture of the distal humerus, with wide separation of the humeral condyles (B). Post-reduction radiographs (**C, D**) showed that the transcondylar screw provided good reduction of the fracture, with restoration of the distal humeral articular surface to a near anatomical condition (D, solid arrow). The single intramedullary pin fixes the proximal fragment to the condylar fragments. The small screws and intramedullary pin assist in providing rotational stability. The tensionband apparatus (C, hollow arrow) repositions and holds the olecranon that was removed to permit exposure of the fracture at the time of surgical reduction.*

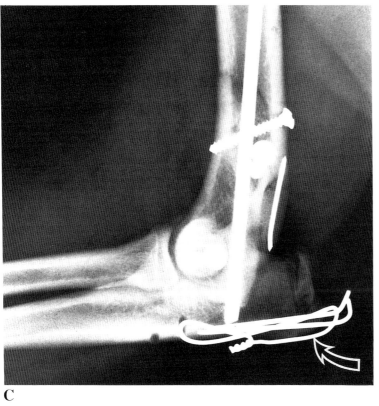

C

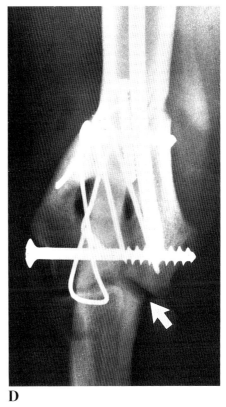

D

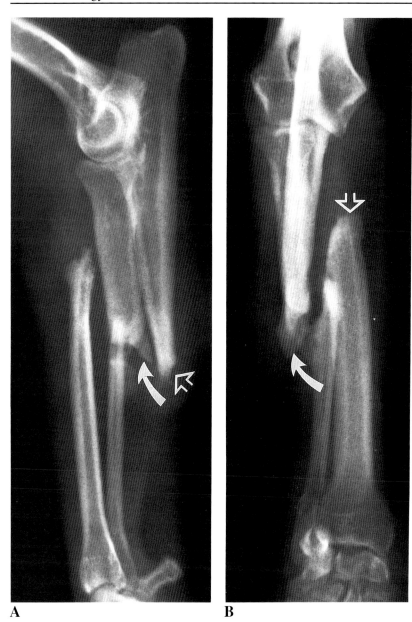

A   B

Figure 4-65.
Radial-ulnar fractures
This mature mix-breed dog had a history of not using the right forelimb for the
previous 6 months, following an injury to the limb. The leg was not painful on
palpation, and yet motion at the suspect fracture site was easy to elicit. The ra-
diographic examination included both elbow and carpal joints. Oblique
midshaft fractures of both radius and ulna were easy to identify. The chronic
nature of the injury was characterized by the widening of the ends of the bone
(referred to as "elephant foot" formation) and by the pseudoarthrosis that had
formed between the proximal radial fragment and the distal ulnar fragment
(solid arrows). No radiographic evidence of any bridging callus formation
was noted and all of the ends of the fracture fragments were smooth and
rounded indicating inactivity. The proximal ulnar and distal radial fragments
were not involved in a healing process nor in the formation of pseudoarthrosis,
and, therefore, had atrophied with "pointing" or "penciling" of the ends of
the bone (hollow arrows). Disuse osteopenia was evident within the distal ra-
dius and ulna and within the carpal bones.

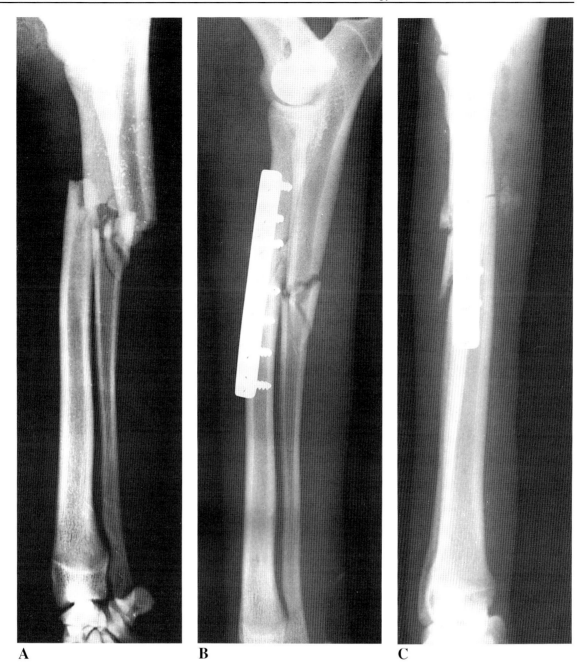

A   B   C

Figure 4-66.
Radial-ulnar fractures.
Badly comminuted radial and ulnar fractures are seen on the lateral radiograph (A). Minimal over-riding of the fragments is noted. Both proximal and distal joints appear not to be involved. Post-reduction radiographs demonstrate stabilization of the radial fracture utilizing a seven-hole plate (B, C). Stabilization of the radial fracture has resulted in a degree of reduction of the ulnar fracture. The free ulnar fragments are left in position near the fracture site to assist in building the callus that will ultimately bridge the fracture site.

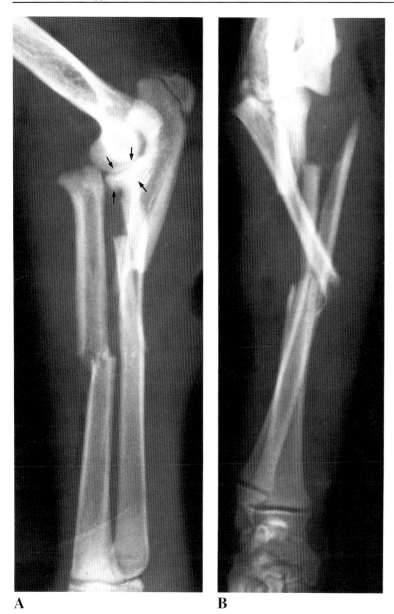

A   B

Figure 4-67.
Radial-ulnar fractures.
A 1-year-old male domestic short-hair cat was attacked by a dog and bit-
*ten in the forelimb. The first radiographic study (**A**, **B**) demonstrated*
particularly severe fractures of the radius and ulna as well as a Type-1
physeal fracture involving the proximal radius, with complete separa-
tion of the proximal epiphysis that is hidden behind the medial coronoid
process of the proximal ulna (arrows). Soft tissue gas indicates the open
*nature of the fracture. Post-reduction radiographs (**C**, **D**) were made 9*
days after reduction and showed alignment of the ulnar fragments; how-
ever, there was no end-to-end apposition of the radial fragments (long
arrows). The last radiographic study showed good healing of the frac-
*tures, 8-months later (**E**, **F**). The remodeling of the fracture callus in this*
cat is remarkable and attests to the healing potential in a skeletally im-
mature patient. Unfortunately there is some cross-healing (synostosis)
between the radius and ulna that limits supination. However, the cat was
able to move the limb without apparent pain.

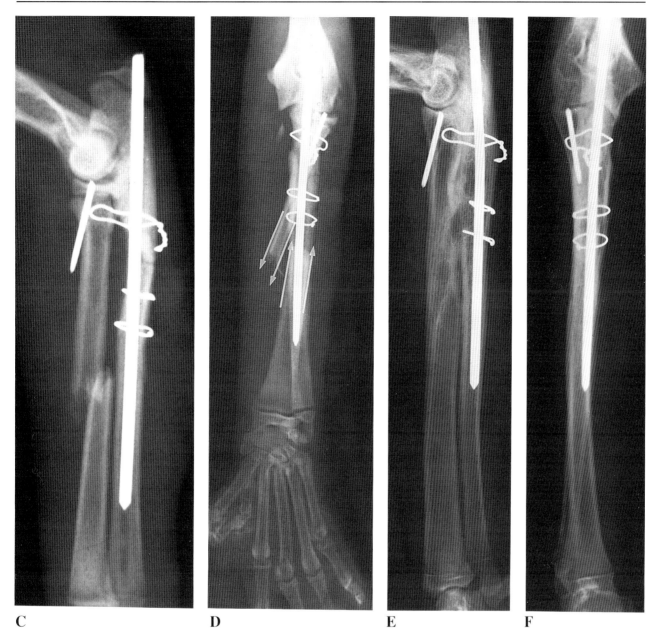

C   D   E   F

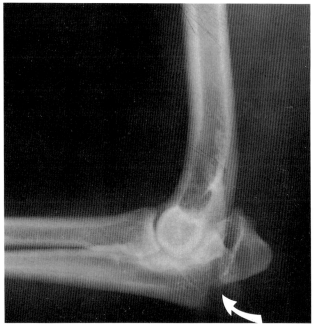

A

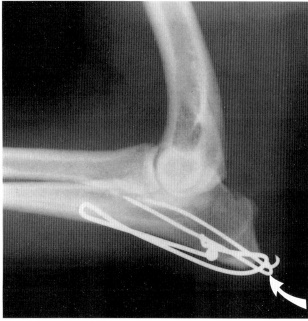

B

Figure 4-68.
Olecranon fracture.
*A mature male Miniature Poodle had fallen and was unable to use the left forelimb after the injury. Radiographs at the time of injury (**A**) showed the avulsion of the olecranon process (arrow). A radiograph made post-reduction (**B**) showed good reduction and stabilization of the fracture fragment utilizing a tension-band wire technique (arrow).*

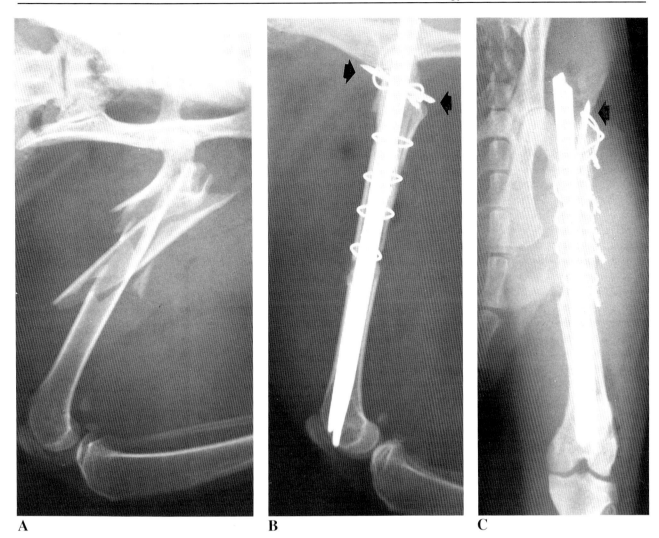

A   B   C

Figure 4-71.
Femoral fracture.
*A comminuted midshaft femoral fracture with several large "butterfly" fragments is seen in a mature cat (**A**). The fracture lines extend proximally and include the greater trochanter. Both hip and stifle joints are unaffected. Excellent reduction is obtained by means of stacked intramedullary pins (**B, C**). Multiple cerclage wires were needed to hold the free cortical fragments in position. A tension-band device (arrows) was used to replace the trochanteric fragment. Notice the sharp fragment borders that indicate that the fracture is of recent origin.*

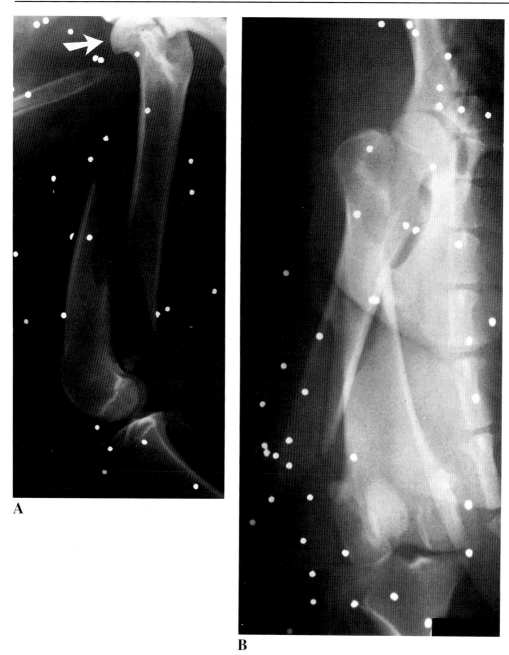

A

B

Figure 4-72.
Femoral fracture.
Radiographs in a mature dog demonstrate an oblique midshaft femoral fracture with marked over-riding of the major fragments (A, B). Note the anteversion position of the femoral head on the lateral view (arrow) that needs to be corrected during fracture stabilization. The presence of metallic shot within the soft tissues is unrelated to the fracture and represents an earlier injury. Post-reduction lateral and craniocaudal radiographs (C, D) demonstrate the use of an intramedullary pin and four full cerclage wires to achieve axial stability. A half-pin Kirschner apparatus was used to achieve rotational stability.

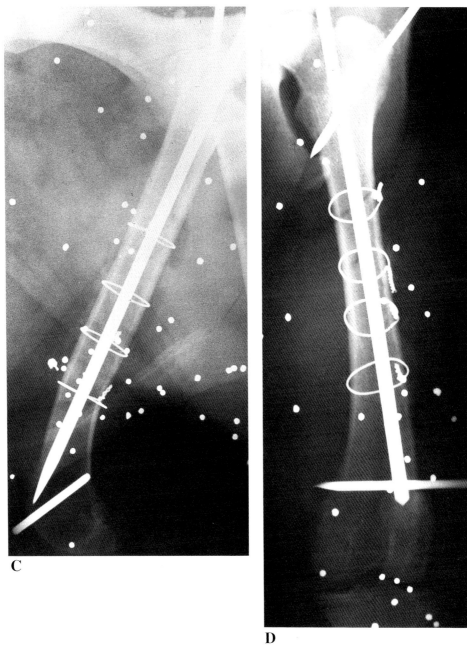

C

D

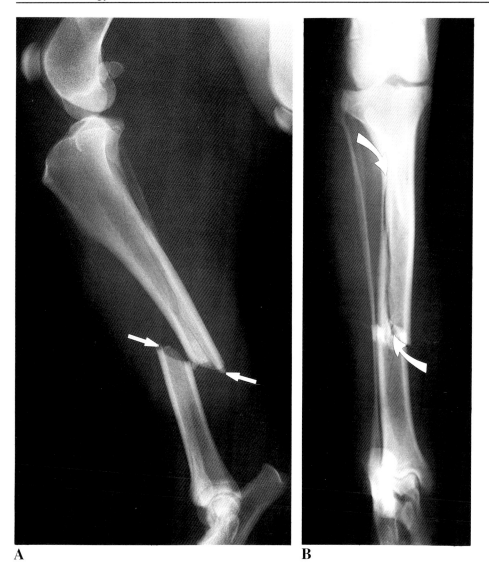

A   **B**

Figure 4-73.
Tibial Fracture.

*A 5-year-old male German Shepherd Dog has a short oblique fracture of the tibia as seen on the lateral view (**A**, straight arrows). However, a most important long fissure line that extended proximally into the metaphyseal region (curved arrows) can only be identified on the caudocranial view (**B**). This is a good example of the danger of only using one radiographic view to determine the nature of the fracture and the type of stabilization that needs to be used for fixation.*

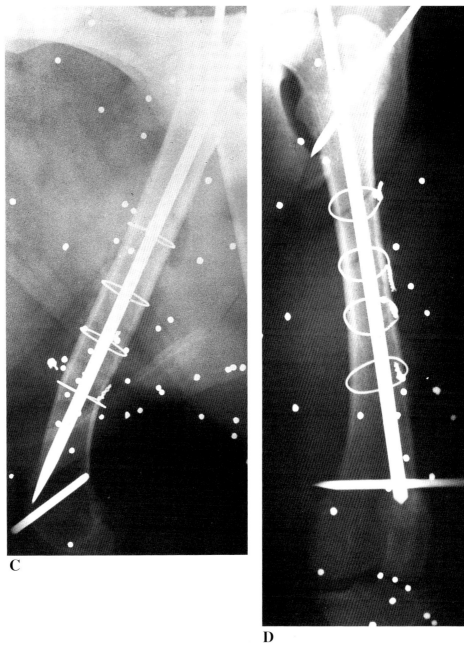

C

D

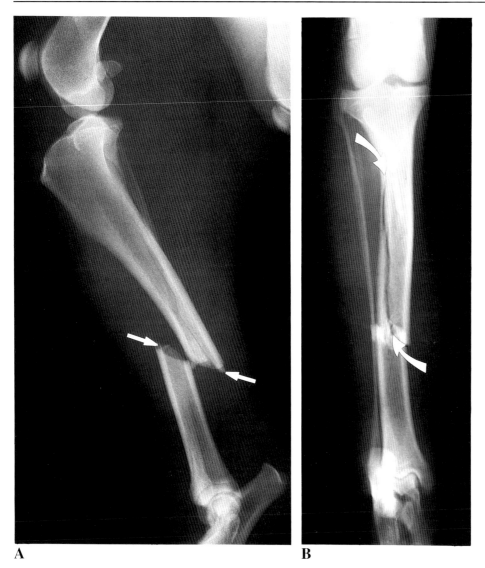

A   **B**

Figure 4-73.
Tibial Fracture.
*A 5-year-old male German Shepherd Dog has a short oblique fracture of the tibia as seen on the lateral view (**A**, straight arrows). However, a most important long fissure line that extended proximally into the metaphyseal region (curved arrows) can only be identified on the caudocranial view (**B**). This is a good example of the danger of only using one radiographic view to determine the nature of the fracture and the type of stabilization that needs to be used for fixation.*

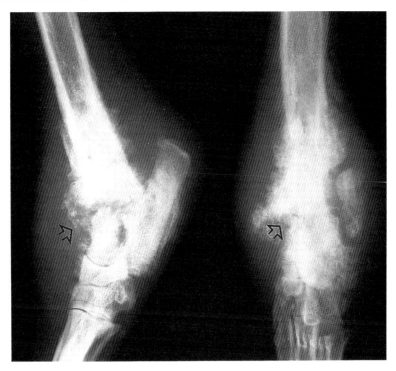

Figure 4-74.
Post-injury osteomyelitis/infectious arthritis.
An 8-year-old female Irish Setter was bitten in the foot by a rattlesnake. The foot became badly swollen and a fistulous tract developed. The foot was curetted and the dog placed on antibiotic therapy. Radiographs of the foot were made 3 months after the original injury. Infectious arthritis (hollow arrows) has destroyed the tibiotarsal joint, and osteomyelitis is evident within the distal tibia and the proximal row of tarsal bones.

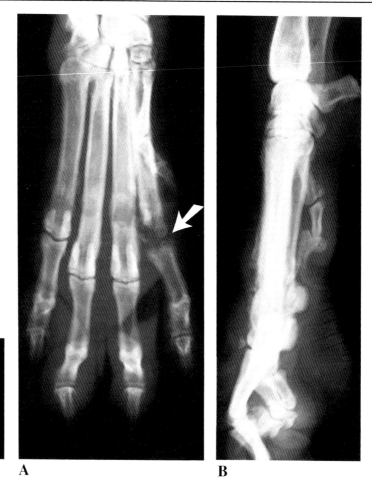

A   **B**

Figure 4-75.
Post-injury osteomyelitis/infectious arthritis.
*A mature Shepherd-cross had his right forefoot caught in a trap overnight. Upon release, the foot was swollen and the soft tissues were cold. Two weeks following the injury, radiographs (**A, B**) demonstrated an area of osteolysis in the distal second metacarpal bone and the adjacent proximal first phalanx (arrow). This pattern of bone destruction associated with a joint space is diagnostic of ostemyelitis and infectious arthritis.*

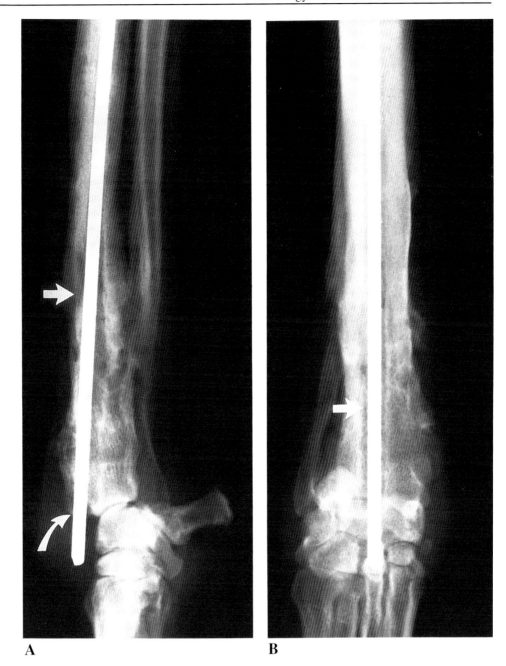

A   **B**

Figure 4-76.
Post-fracture osteomyelitis.
*A radial-ulnar fracture was repaired by means of a single intramedullary pin. Control ra-
diographs were made 4 weeks after surgery (**A, B**) that showed an irregular pattern of callus
formation, with bony bridging between the radius and ulna. A focal radiolucent pattern was
visible around the pin, with apparent draining tracts (straight arrows) strongly suggesting
bone infection. If the pattern of lucency is regular and envelopes the entire pin, osteolysis is
probably due to motion of the pin. Soft tissue swelling at the carpal region also supports the
idea of an inflammatory process; however, the distal position of the tip of the pin might have
influenced this (curved arrow). A joint tap was positive for bacteria and there was a high
white cell count supporting the diagnosis of osteomyelitis.*

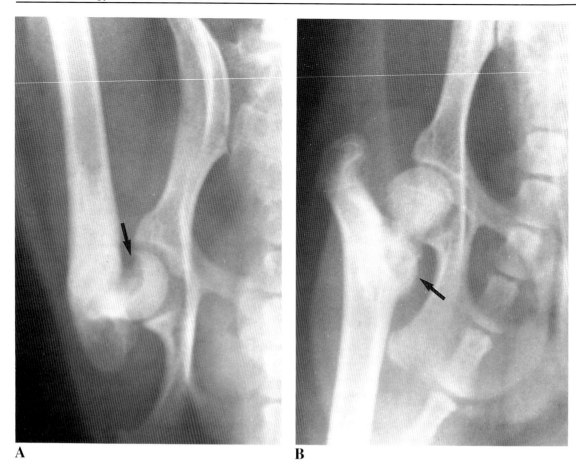

A

B

Figure 4-77.

Post-traumatic aseptic necrosis following capital femoral physeal fracture.

*A Welsh Terrier sustained trauma at 3 months of age resulting in separation of the capital epiphysis from the metaphysis of the right femur (**A**, arrow). Two months later, resorption of the femoral neck had occurred because of a persistent blood supply, but the capital epiphysis had remained unchanged in shape and density because of the lack of a viable blood supply (**B**). Note the new bone formation in the region of the lesser trochanter (arrow). Four months later, the capital epiphysis and proximal femoral neck had lost density through osteoclasia indicating an ingrowth of a new blood supply (**C**). The loss of bone density within the acetabulum (arrow) was the result of disuse osteopenia. Five months later, the capital epiphysis had disappeared along with most of the femoral neck, and there was marked remodelling of the acetabulum with loss of the original cup shape (**D**).*

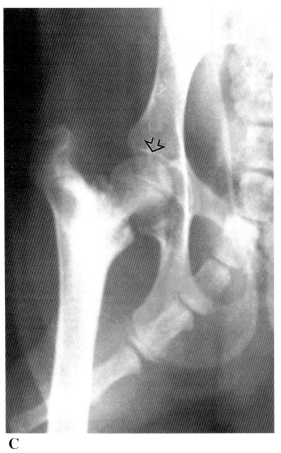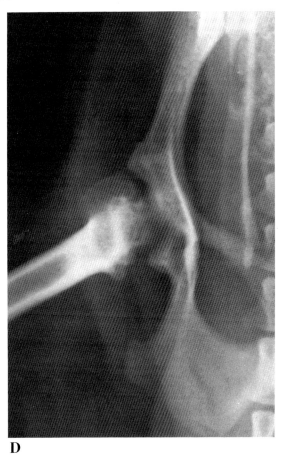

C

D

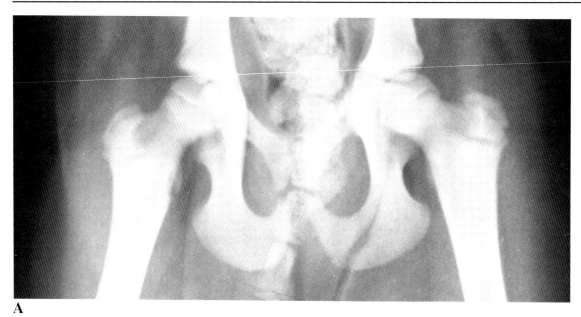

A

Figure 4-78.
Femoral neck fracture with malunion.
This immature dog received a femoral neck fracture of the right hip joint at 12 weeks of age. The radiograph at the time of the original injury did not clearly show a fracture line (A). One month later the fracture site was more easily identified (arrow), and there was resorption of the femoral neck around the fracture and a developing valgus deformity (B). Two months later, the fracture had healed with marked valgus deformity (C, black lines). This injury was thought to be outside the attachment of the joint capsule since the capital epiphysis retained its blood supply. Because of failure to stabilize the fracture, malunion resulted with valgus deformity.

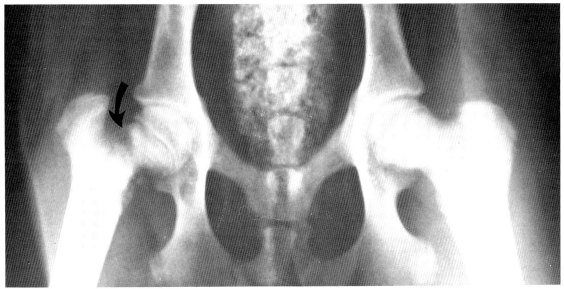

B

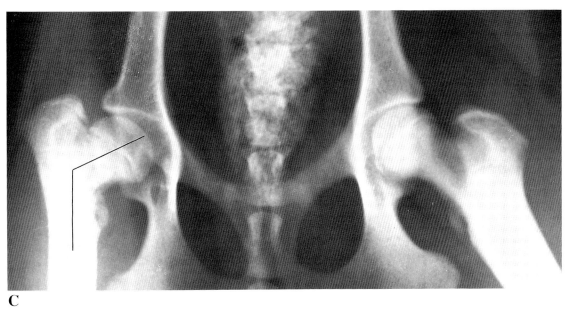

C

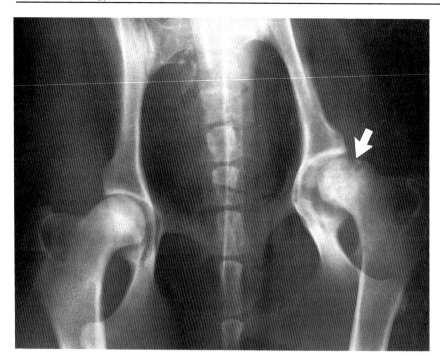
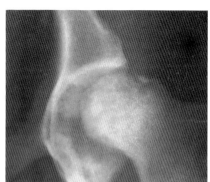

Figure 4-79.
Spontaneous aseptic femoral head necrosis.
In this well-positioned ventrodorsal radiograph of the pelvis of a 9-month-old Poodle it is rather easy to make the comparison of the density and shape of the femoral heads. The mottled appearance of the femoral head on the left (arrow) was due to deposition of new bone together with removal of dead bone tissue. This pattern of repair is referred to as a "creeping substitution". Because of disuse of the limb due to pain, marked soft tissue atrophy was present permitting subluxation of the femoral head. The femoral head will eventually be replaced by viable bony tissue; however, the shape will not be anatomical and secondary arthrosis will develop. Because of the light weight of the dog, the clinical signs were not prominent.

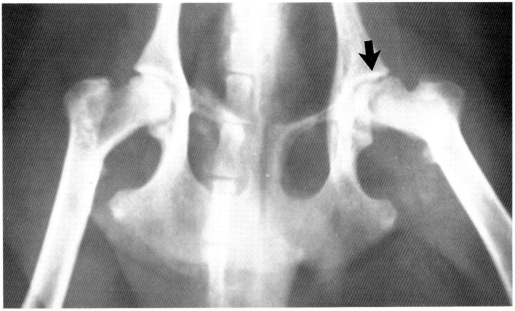

A

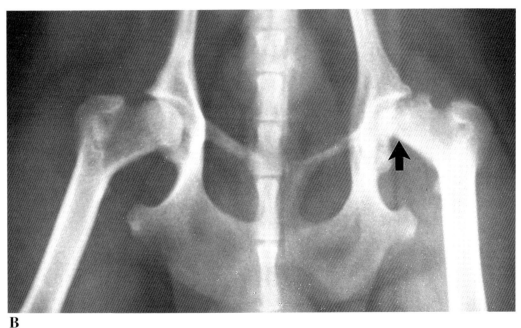

B

Figure 4-80.
Spontaneous aseptic femoral head necrosis.
*Radiographs of a 10-month-old Poodle with left hind limb lameness were made at the time of original entry to the clinic (**A**). The abnormal left femoral head appeared to have suffered from pressure from the acetabular rim (arrow). A second study made 30 days later (**B**), showed more complete remodelling of the femoral head. Secondary arthrosis developed quickly and the dog did not use the limb. Note the arthrosis in the right hip joint that remained essentially unchanged between the two studies. It would appear that the level of aseptic bone necrosis on the right was much less than on the left, or was more efficiently repaired, and that the malformation of the femoral head was therefore less severe on that side resulting in only minimal secondary arthrosis.*

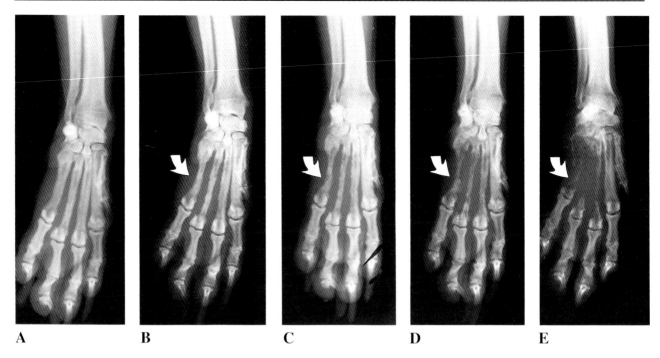

A   B   C   D   E

Figure 4-81.
Post-traumatic osteoporosis.
*A Cairn Terrier was radiographed the first time when he was 11 months of age (**A**) when showing a tendency to not use the left forefoot in a normal manner. Subsequent radiographs were made at 12 (**B**), 13 (**C**), 14 (**D**), and 16 months of age (**E**). These studies showed a gradual disappearance of the 3rd, 4th, and 5th metacarpal bones (arrows). Changes in other bones on the later studies were assumed to be due to disuse osteoporosis. A definitive diagnosis was not possible in this dog, although the changes noted radiographically match the descriptions of post-traumatic osteoporosis.*

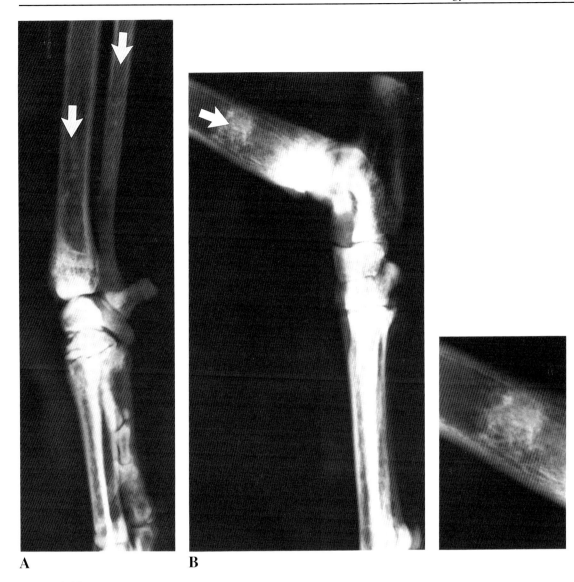

A   **B**

Figure 4-82.
Bone infarcts.
Radiographic changes of medullary densities with "rope-like" patterns are typical for bone infarcts (arrows). The clinical significance of these changes is difficult to ascertain. They are occasionally associated with primary malignant bone tumors, but seem to be of minor clinical importance in other animals.

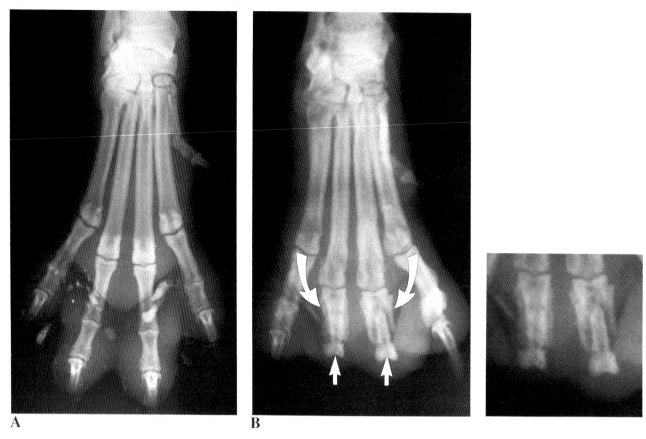

A   B

Figure 4-83.
Trophic bone defect.
This dog was presented to the clinic with a swollen, discolored forefoot after having being outside all night in freezing temperatures. Physical injury to the foot could not be excluded. The first radiograph (A) demonstrated soft tissue swelling with no evidence of bone or joint injury. Radiopaque debris within the soft tissues is easily identified on the radiograph. The second radiograph (B), made 3 weeks later, showed the death and surgical removal of the terminal phalanges of the 4th and 5th digits, with sequestration of the distal portions of the middle phalanges of these digits (straight arrows). The proximal portion of these phalanges show signs of viability as evidenced by the production of new bone (curved arrows) that tends to surround the sequestra.

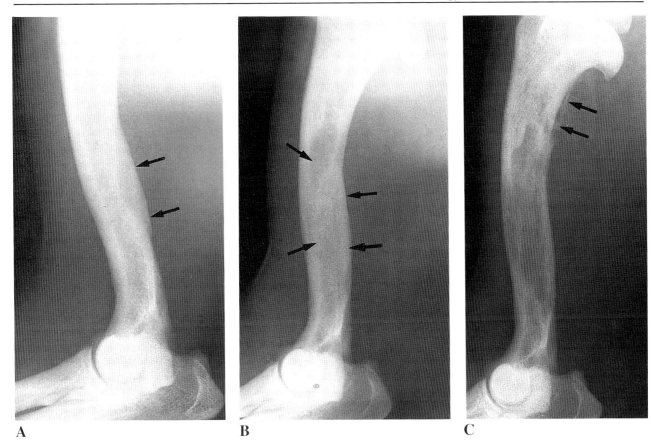

A   B   C

Figure 4-84.
Radium-induced radiation injury.
*Radiographs of the humerus of a male Beagle were made at 6 (**A**), 6.5 (**B**), and 6.6 (**C**) years of age. The first study (A) showed a smooth periosteal reactive bone formation on the caudal cortex, with a small linear cortical lucency (arrows). This lucency increased in size on the second study (B), with additional new bone deposited on the periosteal and endosteal surfaces (arrows). In the last study (C), bone destruction had markedly increased and there was a break in the caudal cortex, with a more aggressive type of periosteal reactive new bone formation (arrows). The leg was amputated because of pain and lameness. Histological diagnosis was that of an osteosarcoma, with a pathological fracture. Multiple pulmonary metastases were present at necropsy, one month later.*

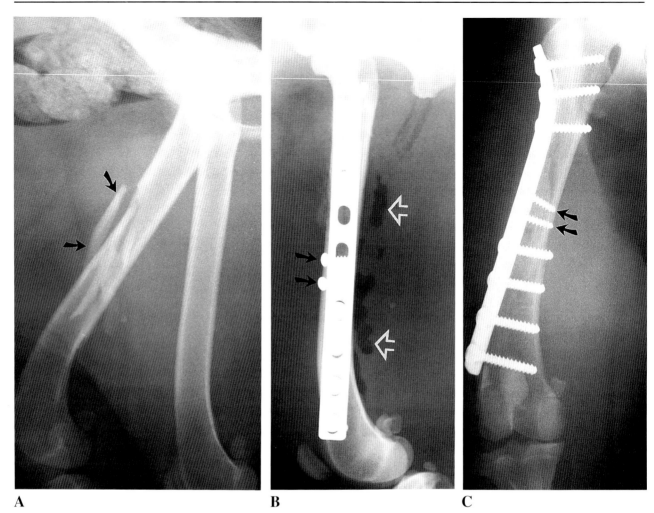

A   **B**   **C**

Figure 4-85.
Use of screws in fracture stabilization.
*A lateral radiograph (**A**) showed a comminuted femoral fracture, with a single large butterfly fragment (arrows). Reduction of the butterfly fragment was obtained by using two lag screws (black arrows) plus 7 other screws that held a neutralization plate in position on the lateral cortical surface (**B, C**). The lateral post-operative radiograph (**B**) showed free air in the soft tissues surrounding the fracture site (hollow white arrows). A drawing of a similar type of fracture stabilization shows the use of two lag screws (arrows) that hold a butterfly fragment in position (**D**).*

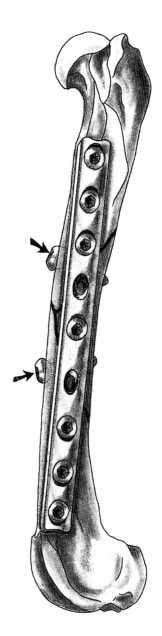

D

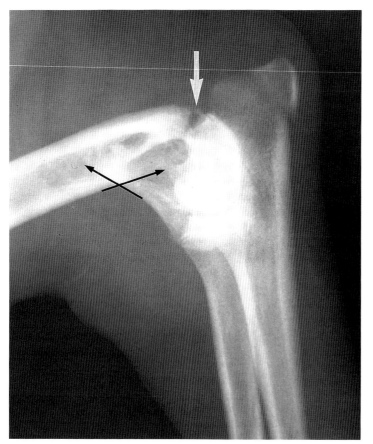

A

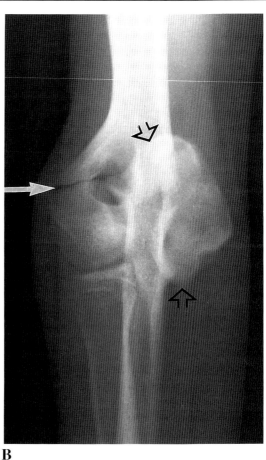

B

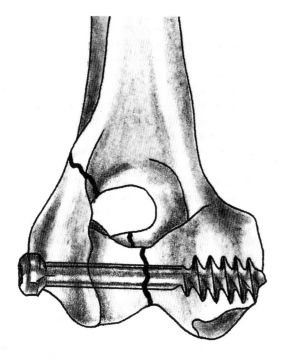

C

Figure 4-86.
Use of cancellous screws in fragment stabilization.
*Lateral (**A**) and craniocaudal (**B**) radiographs of the elbow joint illustrated a typical "Y" type fracture of the distal humerus (solid arrows). The position of the humeral fragments showed marked over-riding, with malaligned cranial cortices (A, long black arrows). The displaced medial condyle of the distal humerus was identified (B, hollow arrows) while the lateral condyle, even though fractured free, had remained in a more anatomically normal position. A drawing (**C**) shows more clearly the use of a partially threaded cancellous screw to stabilize an intra-articular fracture of the lateral humeral condyle.*

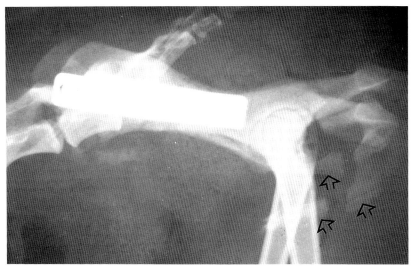

A

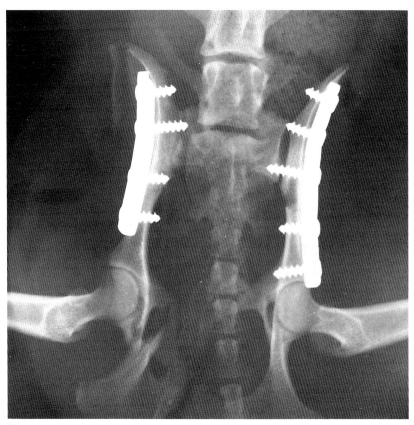

B

Figure 4-87.
Use of contoured plates to stabilize ilial fractures.
*Lateral (**A**) and ventrodorsal (**B**) radiographs show reduction and stabilization of ilial shaft fractures using contoured bone plates. By reduction of the ilial fractures, there has been some realignment of the ischial fragments. Cancellous screws can be selected to a length that they enter the sacrum if luxation of the sacroiliac joint is present. Reduction of fractures of the pubis (arrows) was not attempted. They usually unite by fibrocartilaginous callus. Note that fracture lines do not involve the acetabulae.*

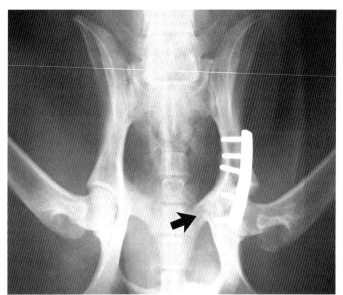

A

Figure 4-88.
Use of contoured plates to stabilize an acetabular fracture.
*Ventral (**A**) and lateral (**B**) radiographs show reduction and stabilization of an acetabular fracture (A, solid arrow) by means of a contoured bone plate. Reduction of the fracture is not anatomical (B, hollow arrow), and post-fracture arthrosis should be expected. A drawing of the pelvis (**C**) depicts the placement of a contoured "finger" plate on the dorsal ridge of the acetabulum.*

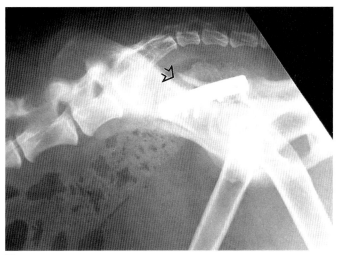

B

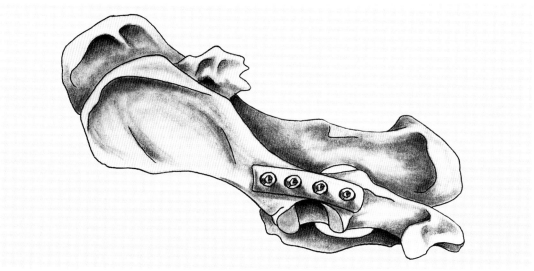

C

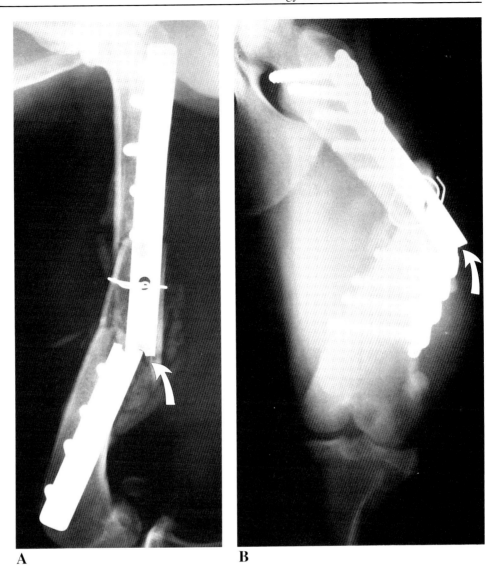

A   B

Figure 4-89.
Fractured plate.
A 1-year-old male Labrador Retriever had a femoral fracture plated 3-weeks earlier but would not bear weight on the limb after two weeks. The dog presented with a swollen limb, hot to touch, which rotated inwardly. The dog had been very active physically after the original fracture treatment. Radiographs showed an 11-hole plate that had fractured through a hole (arrows). The single cerclage wire had remained unchanged in position. The amount of callus formation at the fracture site is typical for fracture healing at 2-3 weeks.

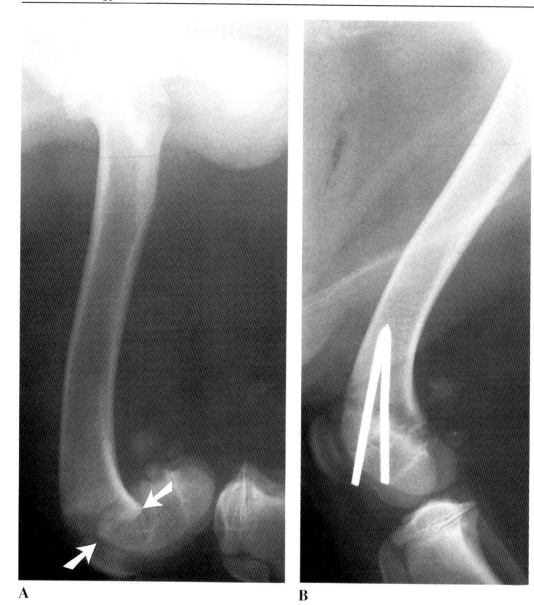

Figure 4-90.
Use of cross pinning.
*A lateral radiograph of the femur showed a Type-I physeal fracture of the distal femur (**A**). The malpositioned distal end of the major fragment is easily identified (arrows). Note the caudal rotation and displacement of the distal bone fragment. Lateral (**B**) and craniocaudal (**C**) radiographs of the femur showed reduction and stabilization of the physeal fracture using 2 cross pins with a small diameter. The apparent medial angulation of the distal femur as seen on the craniocaudal radiograph (C, arrows) is due to positioning of the limb for radiography, and is not real. It is important to understand that positioning of the limb for radiographic examination must be performed very carefully since it greatly influences the presentation of fragment positioning on the radiographs.*
*A craniocaudal drawing (**D**) illustrates stabilization of a Type-I physeal fracture of the distal femur utilizing 2 cross pins.*

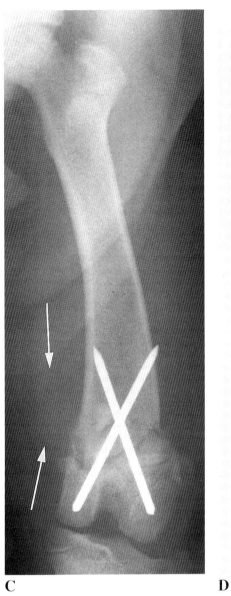

C

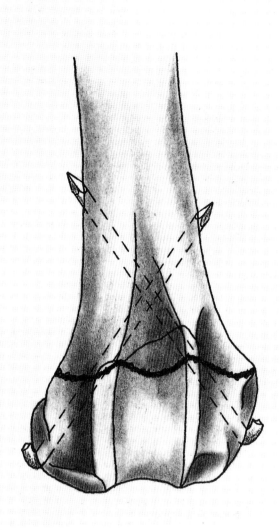

D

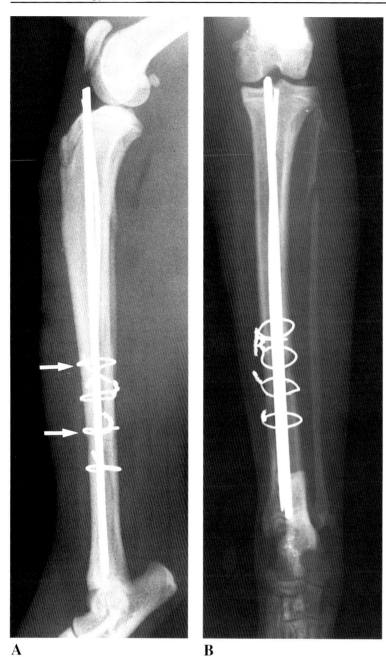

A   **B**

Figure 4-91.
Use of cerclage wires.
*Post-surgical lateral (**A**) and craniocaudal (**B**) radiographs showed successful reduction and stabilization of a distal tibial fracture using 4 full cerclage wires tightly placed (arrows) plus two stacked intramedullary pins. Additional radiographs (**C**, **D**) made 6 weeks post-reduction showed minimal callus formation at the fracture site. Notice that callus formed over the cerclage wires (arrows). Fracture lines could no longer be identified on the latter study. The proximal fibular fracture had healed with a more exuberant callus because of continued motion at the fracture site.*

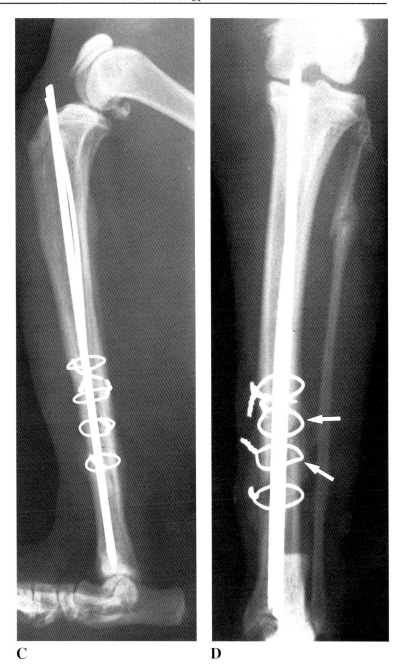

C   D

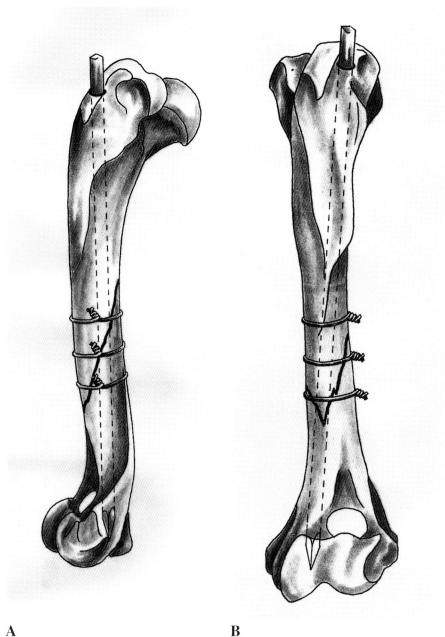

A   **B**

Figure 4-92.
Use of cerclage wires.
*Drawings of lateral (**A**) and craniocaudal (**B**) views illustrate application of an intramedullary pin that is used to achieve axial stabilization of a long oblique humeral fracture plus placement of 3 cerclage wires that insure close fit of the fracture fragments to each other and around the intramedullary pin, thus providing and maintaining rotational stability. The cerclage wires are evenly spaced and tightly encircle the diaphysis so that no motion is possible along the shaft of the bone.*

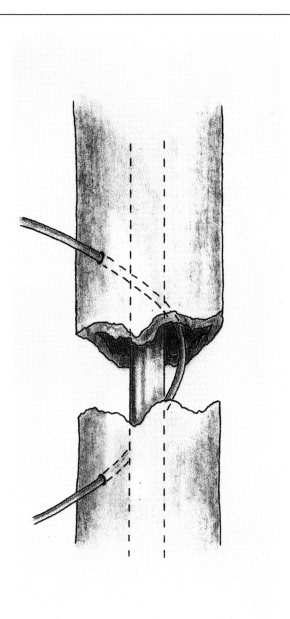

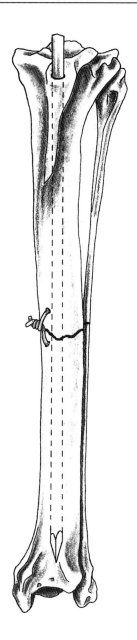

A   B

Figure 4-93.
Use of a hemicerclage wire.
Drawings show the placement of a hemicerclage wire as it enters through the cortex of the proximal fragment, encircles the intramedullary pin, and exits through the cortex of the distal fragment. Used in this way, the wire controls axial movement while the intramedullary pin achieves axial stability in the treatment of a transverse tibial fracture.

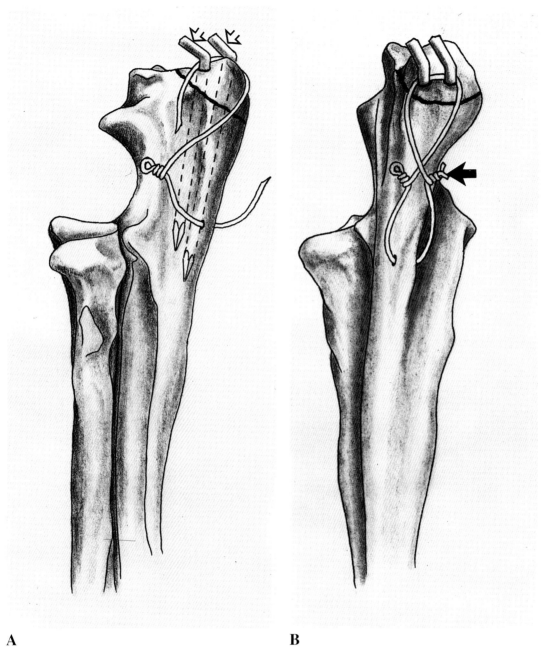

A   **B**

Figure 4-94.
Use of a tension-band wiring technique.
Lateral (A) and caudocranial (B) drawings of the proximal ulna show parallel wires (hollow arrows)
that are placed to provide rotational stability and to reduce shearing forces between the fragments in the
reposition of the tip of the olecranon process of the ulna that was surgically removed. A figure-of-eight
wire is placed on the tension side of the bone and is passed around both ends of the K wires and through
a more distally located drilled hole in the bone, and then tightened (solid arrow).

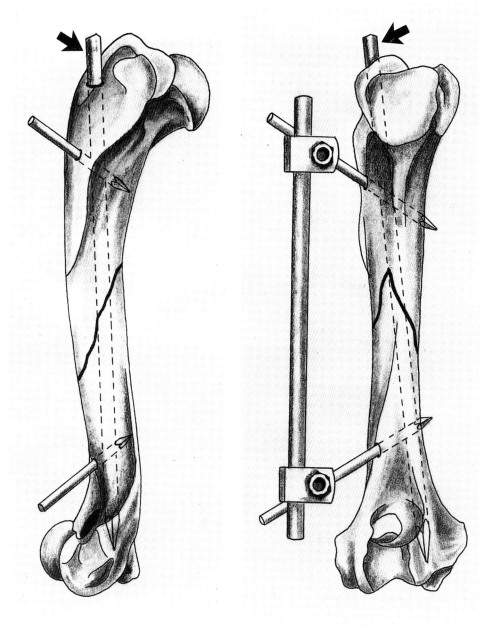

A   **B**

Figure 4-95.
Use of a half-pin Kirschner apparatus.
*Lateral (**A**) and caudocranial (**B**) drawings show reduction and stabilization of an oblique humeral fracture using a half-pin Kirschner apparatus. The Kirschner pins fully penetrate both cortices at an oblique angle to the long axis of the bone. The external fixation device is placed in addition to an intramedullary pin (arrows).*

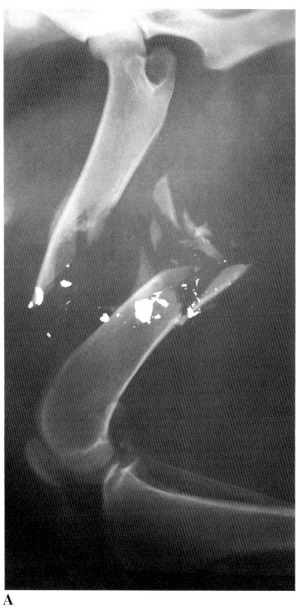

A

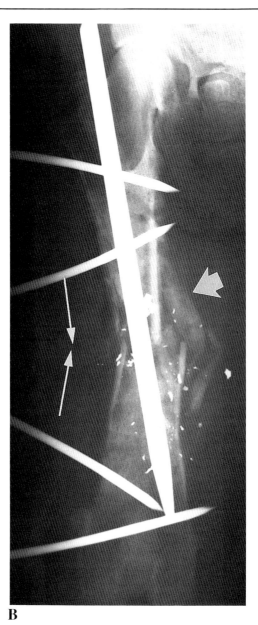

B

Figure 4-96.

Use of a full-pin Kirschner apparatus.

The lateral radiograph (**A**) of a badly comminuted midshaft femoral fracture due to a gunshot injury showed marked separation and over-riding of the fracture fragments. A post-reduction craniocaudal radiograph (**B**) made 4 weeks after the injury showed the use of a full-pin Kirschner device and an intramedullary pin to achieve stability at the fracture site. Minimal lateral deviation of the distal fracture fragments was noticed (long arrows). Callus formation (short arrow) was noted, with expected loss of density of the fracture fragments. It was difficult to judge the degree of callus formation because the addition of a cancellous graft at the time of surgery created a pattern of bone density. The graft adds density at the fracture site and makes the callus formation appear more progressive than it actually is. A craniocaudal drawing (**C**) of the femur illustrates the application of a full-pin Kirschner apparatus to help achieve axial stabilization of a femoral fracture while use of an intramedullary pin produces angular or axial stabilization.

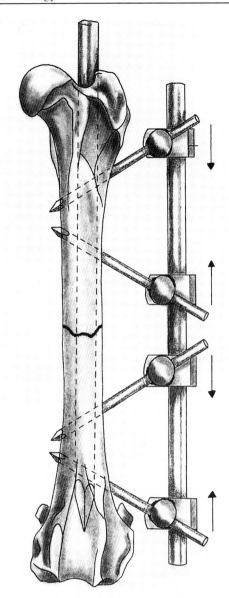

C

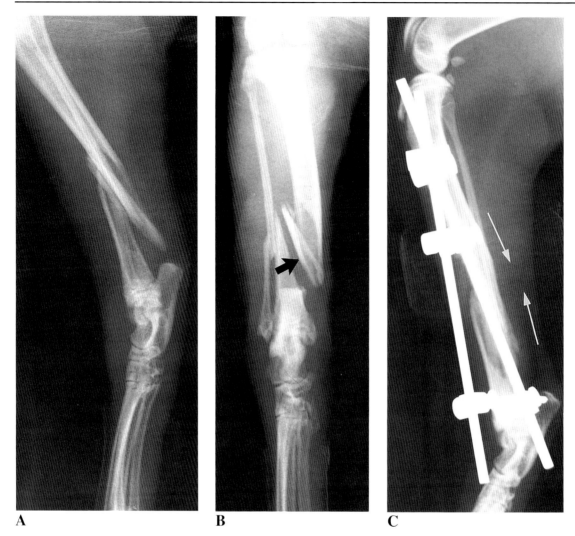

A   B   C

Figure 4-97.
Use of a full-pin Kirschner apparatus.
*Lateral (**A**) and craniocaudal (**B**) radiographs of the right hind leg of a kitten show a long oblique distal tibial fracture with one large butterfly fragment (arrow). A simple fibular fracture is also present. Lateral (**C**) and craniocaudal (**D**) radiographs were made following reduction and stabilization of the tibial fracture using a full-pin Kirschner apparatus. Because of the distal location of the fracture, only one pin could be placed in the distal fragment. Minimal lateral and cranial angulation of the distal fragment was noted (long arrows), neither of which is probably of importance in this patient. A craniocaudal radiograph (**E**) was made 8 weeks laters showing good callus formation that bridged the fracture sites in both bones. A drawing (**F**) of a craniocaudal view shows stabilization of a comminuted tibial fracture using a full-pin Kirschner apparatus.*

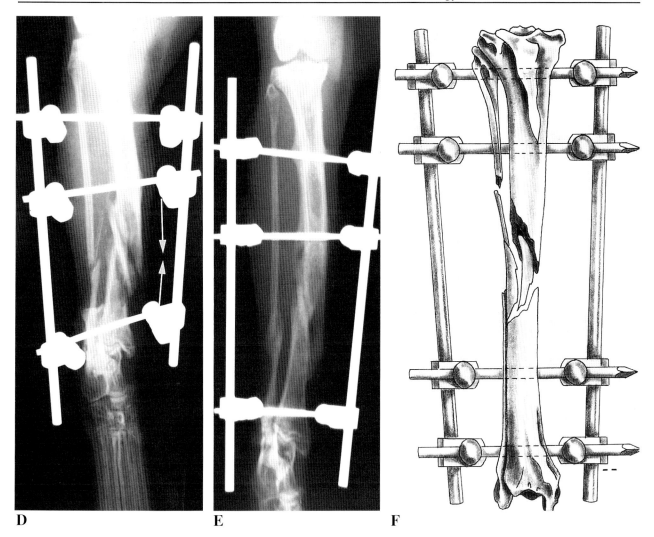

D   **E**   **F**

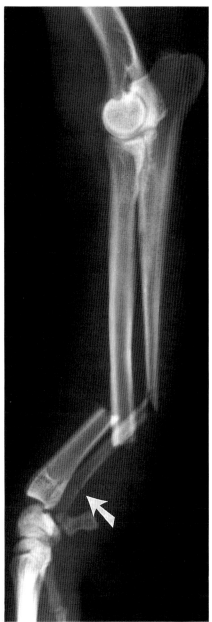

A

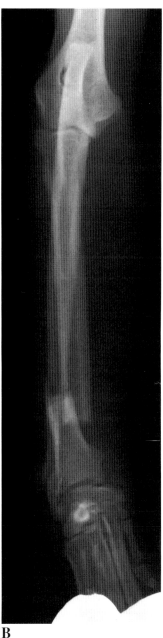

B

Figure 4-98.

Use of intramedullary fixation devices.

Lateral (**A**) *and craniocaudal* (**B**) *radiographs of a front limb showed transverse fractures of the radius and ulna, with overriding and angulation of the fragments. Notice the second ulnar fracture just proximal to the styloid process (A, arrow). Lateral* (**C**) *and craniocaudal* (**D**) *radiographs were made 30 days after stabilization of the radial fracture using a single intramedullary pin. Early signs of callus formation were more prominent in the ulna than in the radius. The delay in fracture healing of the radius was probably due to a combination of compromised extramedullary blood supply: a result of the original soft tissue trauma and the destruction of the intramedullary blood supply by the placement of the intramedullary pin. The protruding tip of the pin (D, arrow) caused subluxation of the radiocarpal joint that will certainly induce post-traumatic joint disease at a later stage. In addition, a very important finding was the external rotation of approximately 90 degrees of the distal fragments. While the intramedullary pin had provided axial stabilization, rotational stabilization that is necessary for this type of fracture had not been provided. A drawing* (**E**) *of a craniocaudal view illustrates the use of a straight Steinmann pin that supplies axial stability to a transverse radial fracture. The pin enters the distal radius on the dorsolateral aspect and its proximal end lodges in the proximal metaphysis. It is usually not necessary to stabilize the ulnar fracture.*

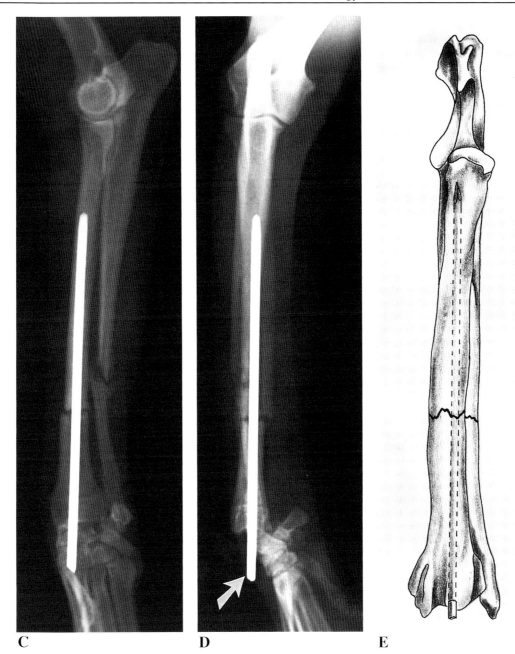

C   D   E

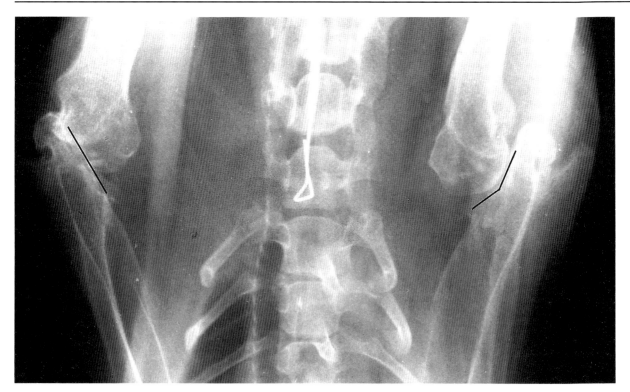

Figure 4-99.
Bilateral chronic shoulder luxations.

As a result of chronic secondary deforming arthrosis both shoulder joints show marked remodeling of the glenoid cavities (black lines) and humeral heads. It is often difficult to ascertain whether lesions like this are post-traumatic or the result of a developmental or congenital anomaly. If lesions appear to have bilateral symmetry, it is easier to assume a congenital or developmental etiology. When shoulder lesions are present in a symmetric way as with this dog, clinical signs are often hidden since both shoulder joints hurt.

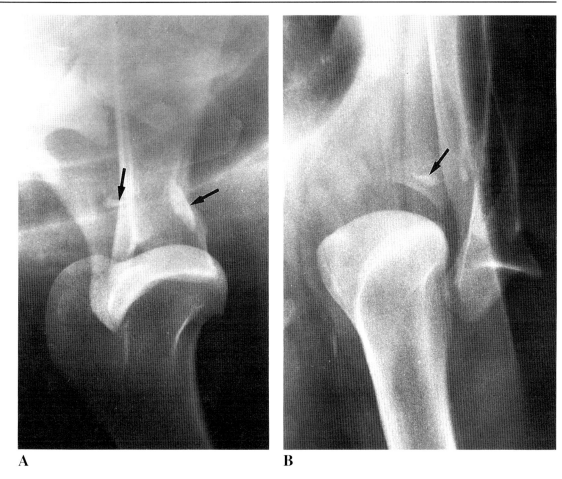

A   **B**

Figure 4-100.
Fracture-luxation of a shoulder joint.
*Lateral (**A**) and caudocranial (**B**) radiographs of a shoulder joint after traumatic injury demonstrated medial luxation of the humeral head. The multiple fracture fragments (arrows) probably originated from the rim of the glenoid cavity and suggest that reduction of the luxation will not be easy.*

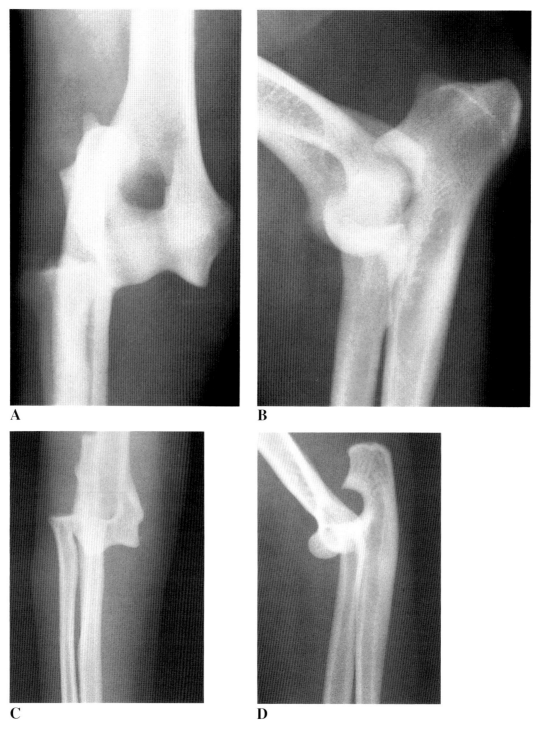

A

B

C

D

Figure 4-101.
Elbow joint luxation.
*A 3-year-old male Collie was hit by a car and suffered a luxated right elbow joint (**A**, **B**). A 3-year-old female Siamese cat returned home, with a lame left forelimb (**C**, **D**). With this kind of injury, it is always important to accurately evaluate the radiographs for signs of any congenital or developmental anomaly that might have predisposed the elbow to luxate. It is also important to examine for fracture fragments or injury to the articular surfaces. In both instances, it may be difficult to achieve permanent reduction of the luxation. It is important to know that with injuries of this type, without evidence of articular surface injury, immediate reduction of the luxation usually results in a near-normal joint without development of appreciable secondary joint disease.*

Figure 4-102.
Antebrachiocarpal luxation.
The injury to the antebrachiocarpal joint in this cat is best evaluated by stressing the foot laterally (arrows) or medially to demonstrate the degree of maximum instability. It is obvious that this painful procedure is best performed after the patient has been sedated. There is little danger in creating additional injury to the joints. In this case, no fracture lines are seen in association with the luxation.

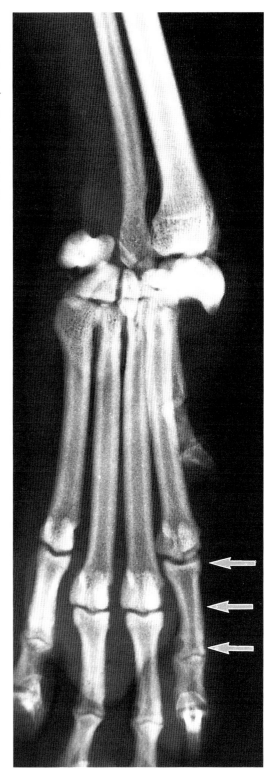

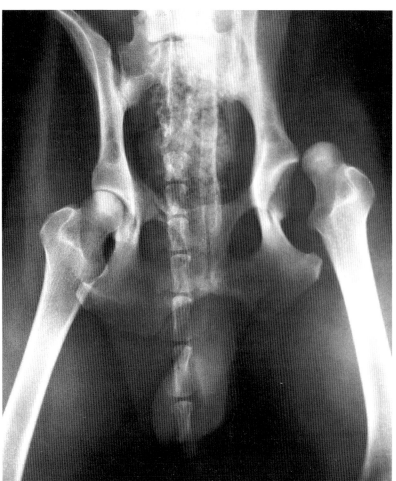

A

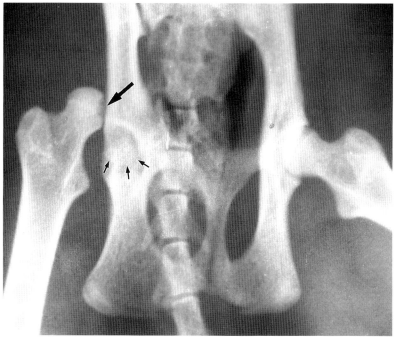

B

Figure 4-103.
Coxofemoral luxations.
Luxation of the left hip joint in a dog (**A**) is without associated fractures, while the luxation of the right hip joint in a cat (**B**) has an avulsion fracture from the femoral head (large arrow) that will complicate reduction. The fracture fragment is represented by an increased density within the acetabulum (small arrows).

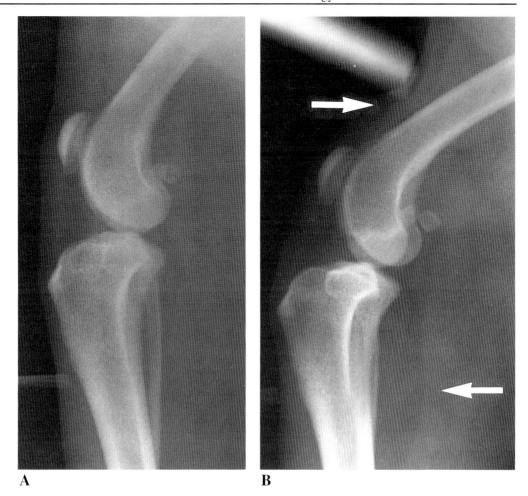

A   **B**

Figure 4-104.
Stifle joint subluxation.
In this 2-year-old female Doberman Pinscher (Doberman), the neutrally positioned radiograph
*(**A**) presented a near-normal stifle joint, while the stress radiograph (**B**) showed marked instabil-*
ity, with cranial displacement of the tibia (arrows). Rupture of the cranial cruciate ligament per-
mitted cranial displacement of the tibia that was demonstrated radiographically. On radiographs
of acutely injured joints, many times no secondary bony changes will be found but joint effusion
may be evident.

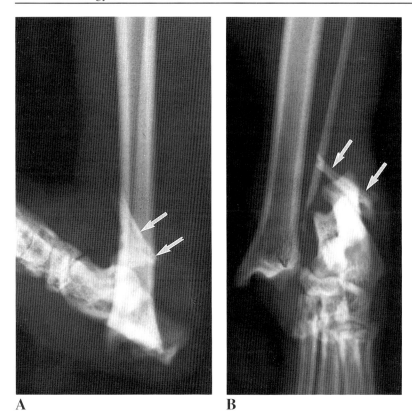

A   B

Figure 4-105.
Tibiotarsal fracture-luxation.
Acute trauma to a 2-year-old male Persian cat with an injury to the hindlimb resulted in a fracture of the lateral malleolus (arrows) that permitted complete luxation of the tibiotarsal joint. Evaluation of soft tissue trauma is important in assessing the degree of injury to the joint. In this cat, tearing of both collateral ligaments had occurred.

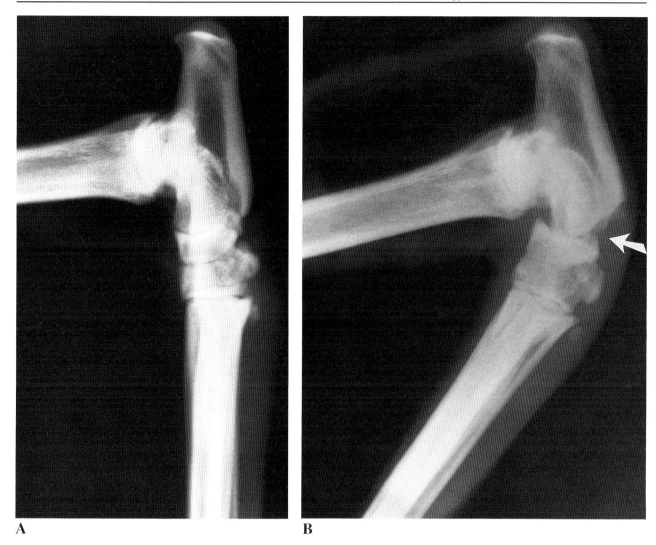

A   B

Figure 4-106.
Proximal intertarsal luxation.
Acute trauma to this 6-year old-male Greyhound occurred during racing and resulted in injury to the hindlimb. While the location of the injury was easily determined on physical examination, radiographs made in a neutral position were thought to be normal (A). However, when the digits were stressed in a hyperextended position (B), a proximal intertarsal luxation due to extensive soft tissue trauma was easily identified (arrow).

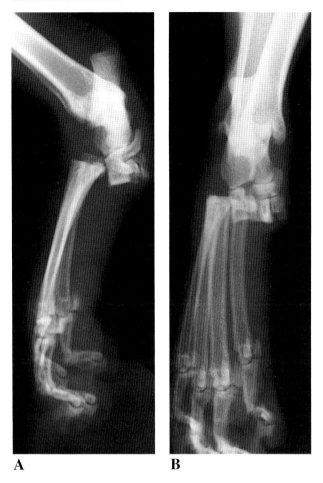

A   B

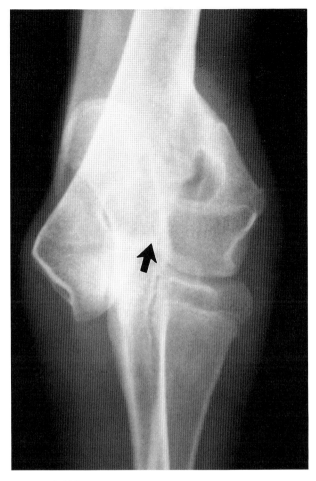

Figure 4-107. **Tarsometatarsal luxation.**
Acute trauma to a 4-year-old male domestic short-haired cat resulted in complete separation of the tarsometatarsal joint, with marked overriding of the bones. Soft tissue injury must be extensive to permit this degree of bone displacement. It is interesting that an injury of this type occurred without associated fracture(s).

Figure 4-108.
Intra-articular fracture.
A lateral epicondylar humeral fracture healed with that fragment of bone malpositioned proximally. This resulted in severe malformation of the articular surfaces of the elbow joint, with development of secondary post-traumatic arthrosis. Anatomical reduction of intra-articular fractures is absolutely necessary to avoid secondary arthrosis. However, the younger the patient, the more repair the cartilaginous surfaces can accomplish, even with malpositioning of the fragments.

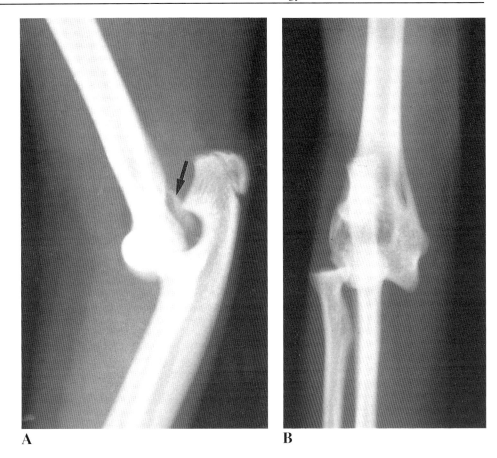

A   B

Figure 4-109.
Acute fracture-luxation of an elbow joint.
*In this cat, there is an extra-articular fracture of the medial epicondyle of the humerus (arrow) at the point of attachment of the carpal flexor tendons (**A**), in addition to a lateral luxation of the radius and ulna (**B**). The fracture indicates a more severe degree of soft-tissue injury that will probably make an attempt at closed reduction of the lesion much more difficult.*

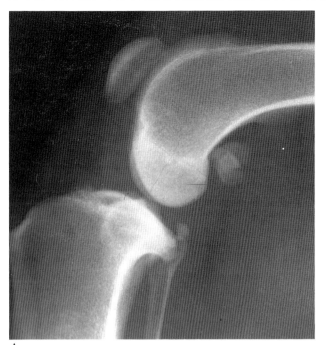

A

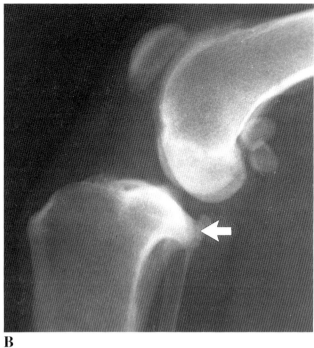

B

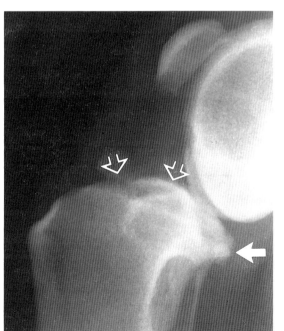

C

Figure 4-110.

Post-traumatic arthrosis.

*This series of radiographs was made of a 9-year-old male mixed-breed dog that injured the right stifle joint during jumping, 5 months earlier. The dog began to reuse the leg at the time of the first study (**A**). The second study (**B**) was made 3 months later when the dog still used the leg, but in an incorrect manner. The final study (**C**) was made 10 months after the first study. This sequence of films shows the progression of joint instability as a result of cranial cruciate ligament injury, and the development of secondary joint disease (arthrosis). Notice the progression in cranial displacement of the proximal tibia (solid arrows) due to rupture of the cranial cruciate ligament as well as the new bone that formed at the attachment site of this ligament on the tibial plateau (hollow arrows).*

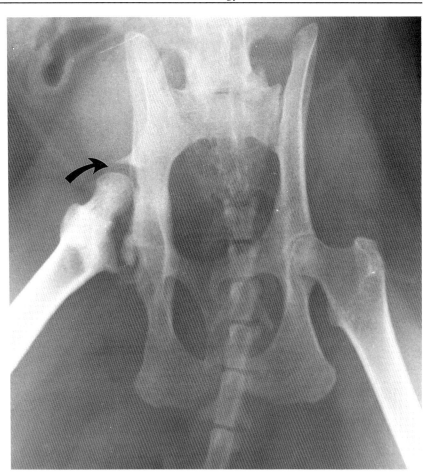

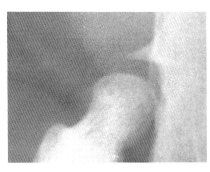

Figure 4-111.
Post-traumatic arthrosis.
A ventrodorsal radiograph of the pelvis of a 4-year-old male cat, with chronic minimal lameness in the right hip joint, demonstrated formation of a pseudoarthrosis following luxation of the femoral head (arrow). Notice the remodeling of the acetabulum with flattening of the original acetabular cup. The new joint usually forms in this location because the femoral head luxates cranially and dorsally, and rests against the shaft of the ilium. The only surgical treatment for this condition, at this time, is a resection of the femoral head and neck, if felt to be necessary at all. However, since cats are usually not required to perform athletically, and usually tolerate the lameness and pain associated with the pseudoarthrosis well, the lesion is often treated conservatively.

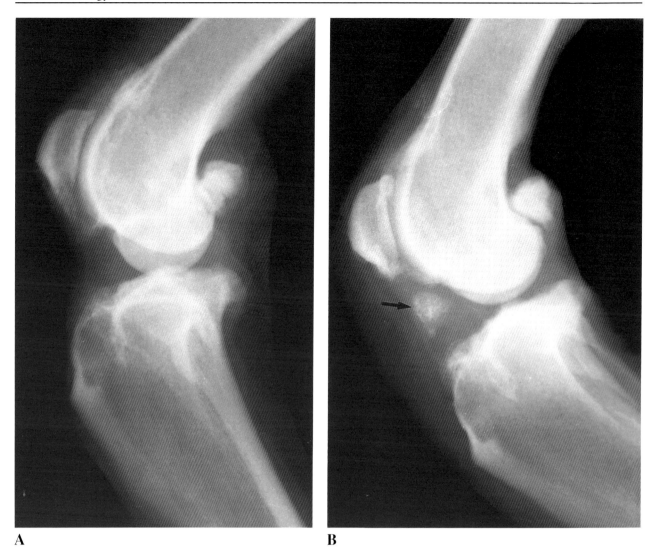

A   B

Figure 4-112.
Chronic joint disease, with free joint body.
*A lateral radiograph of the stifle joint in a 6-year-old Boxer revealed chronic degenerative joint disease (**A**). According to the owner, the dog had been healthy and without complaints until a recent injury when it fell and became acutely lame. The lameness was accentuated because of a traumatic injury superimposed over chronic joint disease. The second study made 6 months later (**B**) showed a free joint body (arrow) that may have been due to an avulsion fracture fragment, synovial osteochondroma, or mineralization of a cartilaginous fragment.*

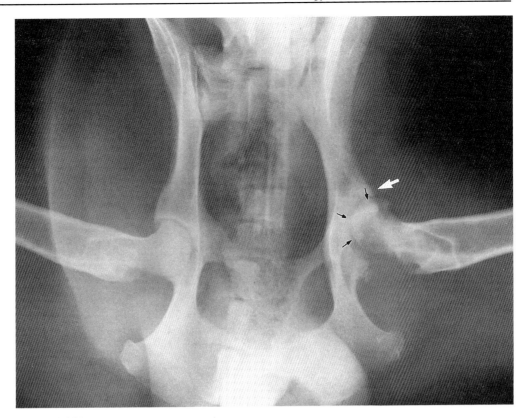

Figure 4-113.
Post-traumatic septic arthritis.
A ventrodorsal view of the pelvis in a 2-year-old male German Shepherd Dog was made follow-ing a suspected left sided coxofemoral luxation several weeks earlier. Lameness was due to pain at first, but became more of a mechanical nature later. At the time of radiography, the dog did not bear weight on the limb. The femoral head was luxated dorsally (small arrows). Both the femoral head and the acetabulum showed loss of bone density possibly due to disuse. Osteopenia was especially evident in the femoral head and neck. Notice also the marked soft tissue atrophy, probably due to disuse. A ridge of newly formed bone was present on the ilium (large arrow). It is important to consider the possibility of infectious arthritis in an animal of this type, and not limit a diagnosis to that of secondary joint disease due to hip dysplasia or to post-traumatic arthrosis. A major radiographic change with infection is the loss of bone density in combination with some new bone formation that presents without a definite pattern. Arthrocentesis is important as a diagnostic test to confirm the diagnosis of infectious arthritis.

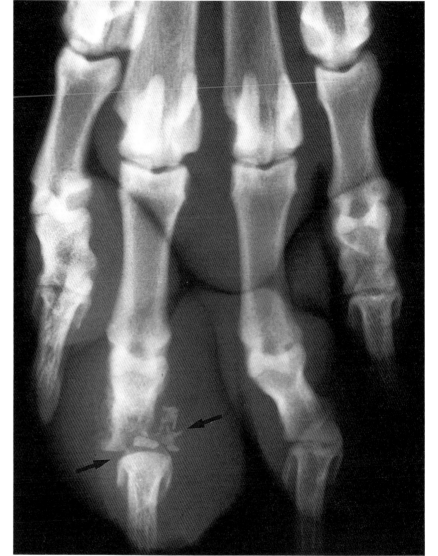

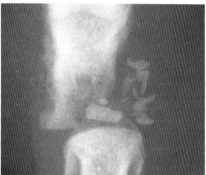

Figure 4-114.
Post-traumatic osteomyelitis and infectious arthritis.
This 5-year-old female Great Dane suffered an injury to the foot that became infected. When radiographed, the foot was swollen and inflamed, and the distal interphalangeal joint of the 4th digit had the radiographic characteristics of an infectious arthritis and osteomyelitis of the second phalanx (arrows). The joint involved space is collapsed. In many cases, the clinical history of a patient like this is incomplete and the soft tissue injury that would have been helpful in achieving the diagnosis of inflammation has healed by the time the patient is presented for examination.

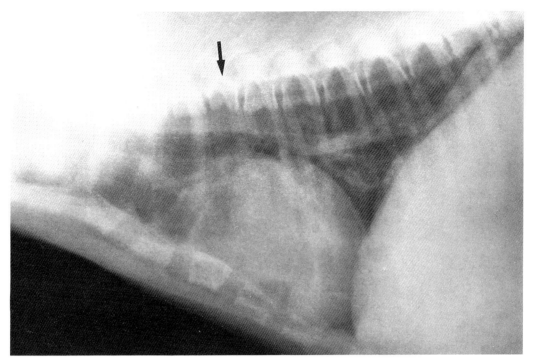

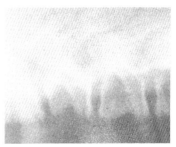

Figure 4-115.
Pathologic fracture of the thoracic spine.

The body of the 5th thoracic vertebral segment was fractured (arrow) in this 6-month-old male kitten. The lack of density in the vertebral bodies suggested a generalized bone disease. Examination of the kitten's diet revealed it to be high in phosphorus and low in calcium resulting in nutritional secondary hyperparathyroidism.

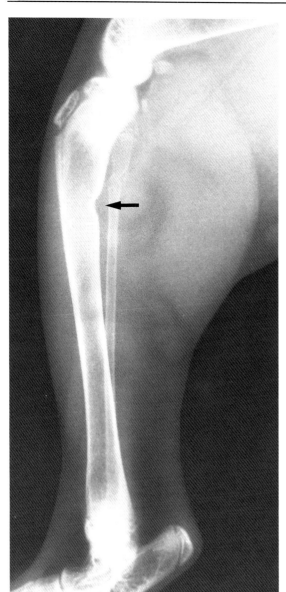

Figure 4-116.
Pathological fracture in a tibia.
Folding fractures (arrow) are characteristic of weakened bone that bends rather than breaks completely with minimal trauma. In this cat, many bones were fractured due to nutritional secondary hyperparathyroidism. The width of the cortical shadows may be less than normal, but this may be difficult to ascertain unless there is a normal litter mate or control cat with which to compare.

Figure 4-117.
Pathological fractures.

*A 3-month-old male Afghan hound jumped down from a 1-meter height, and was immediately lame. A survey skeletal radiographic study was performed. Radiographs of the right (**A**) and left (**B**) forelimbs showed: (1) generalized loss of bone density, with thin cortices, (2) focal increase in bone density in the distal radius and ulna (arrows), and in the midshaft region of the metacarpal bones at the sites of fracture repair (arrows), and (3) altered architecture at the sites of fracture repair due to malunion.*

The thin cortices and loss of cancellous bone were typical of nutritional secondary hyperparathyroidism. The focal increase in bone density was due to the callus formation at the sites of the pathological fractures, with resulting altered architecture in the long bones. Notice that the areas of greatest bone density were present at the site of the fracture callus of the malunion fractures, at the metaphyses where bone growth occurs (hollow arrows), at the periphery of the epiphyses where bone develops from the epiphyseal growth cartilage (hollow arrows), and at the periphery of the small carpal bones (hollow arrows). This suggests that endochondral ossification is occurring at a normal or near-normal rate at physeal plates, epiphyses, small carpal bones as well as at the fracture sites. However, bone tissue once formed does not remain but undergoes osteoclasia in an effort to maintain a normal blood calcium level.

This dog had nutritional secondary hyperparathyroidism, with pathological fractures.

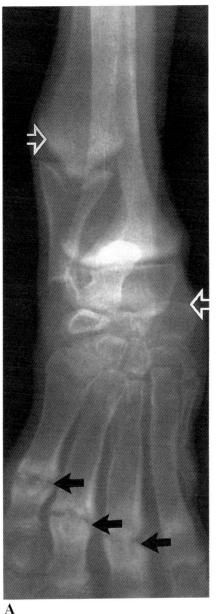

A

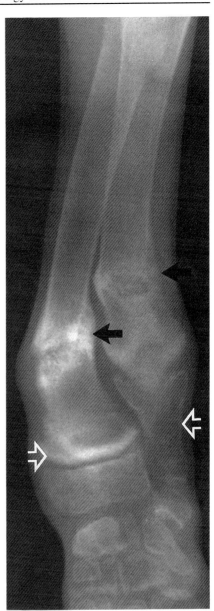

B

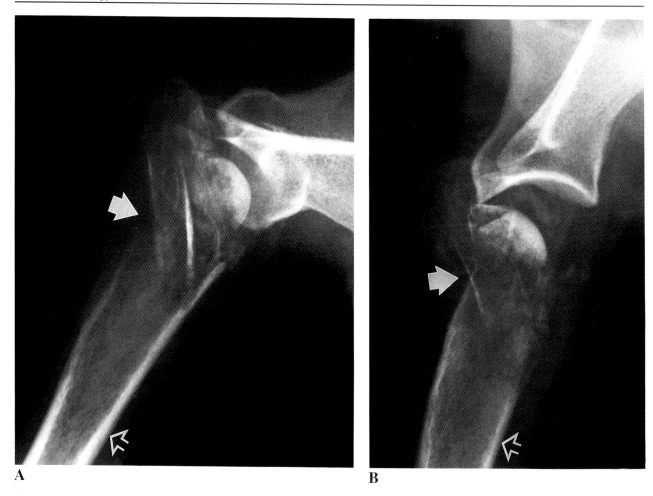

A   **B**

Figure 4-118.
Pathological fracture.
In a 4-year-old male mixed-breed dog, a pathological fracture (solid arrows) in the proximal humerus led to marked deformity of the bone. Notice that the cortex in the middle of the humerus and the scapula is of near-normal density (hollow arrows). This finding excludes the possibility of generalized bone disease, and suggests instead a primary bone lesion such as a primary malignant bone tumor (osteosarcoma, fibrosarcoma, chondrosarcoma, or hemangiosarcoma) or secondary metastatic bone tumor. An inflammatory bone lesion rarely destroys bone to the extent that it fractures. Biopsy was necessary to confirm the diagnosis in this patient, but malignant disease was already strongly suspected. The histopathologic diagnosis was hemangiosarcoma.

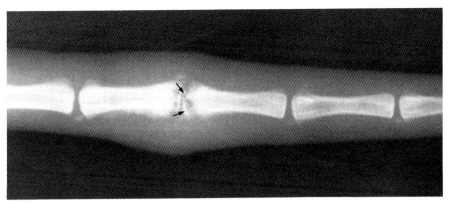

A

Figure 4-119.
Soft tissue swelling.

In a 1-year-old male domestic short-hair cat, soft tissue swelling on the tail was noted (A, B), with collapse of the intervertebral disc space and endplate destruction (arrows) of the underlying caudal vertebrae. The soft tissue swelling on the tail that proved to be centered around a traumatically induced discospondylitis had called attention to this region. Careful examination of the radiographs shows small dense fragments of cortical bone at the site of the disc space that are indicative of bone sequestration.

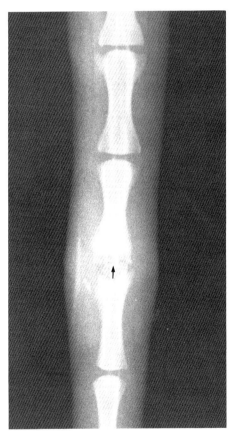

B

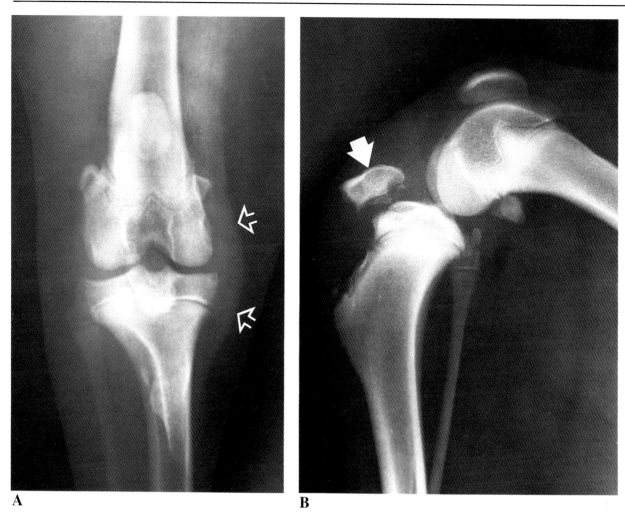

A   B

Figure 4-120.
Soft tissue swelling.
*In a 6-month-old puppy, the stifle joint was greatly swollen (**A**, hollow arrows) following an avulsion fracture of the tibial crest (**B**, solid arrow). Often an abnormal soft tissue mass is detected on physical examination, but radiographic examination is necessary to detect the cause of this soft tissue swelling.*

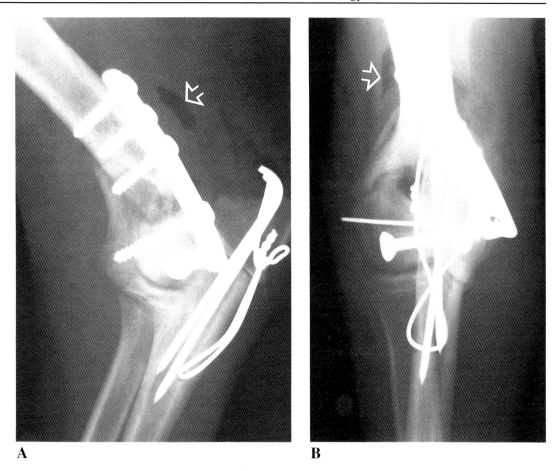

A

B

Figure 4-121.
Soft tissue gas.
Lateral (**A**) *and craniocaudal* (**B**) *radiographs of a post-surgical elbow show that an olecranon osteotomy has been performed as part of a surgical repositioning and stabilization of distal humeral fractures. The intra-articular fracture has been stabilized with a cancellous screw and a single K wire. A neutralization plate has been used along the medial supracondylar ridge to reduce the metaphyseal fracture. The gas within the soft tissues (hollow arrows) can be expected in a post-operative patient, and has no clinical significance.*

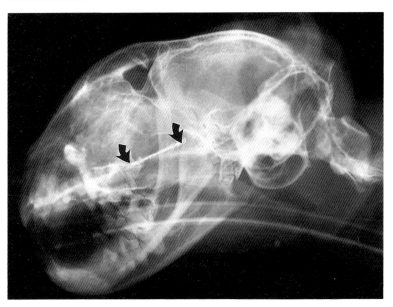

Figure 4-122.
Radiopaque foreign body.
A 6-year-old male cat had a history of chronic nasal discharge for several years. Radiographs were made of the head that demonstrated a metallic foreign body (arrows) in the nasopharynx, with the size and shape of a sewing needle. After removal of the foreign body, the clinical signs disappeared.

Figure 4-123.
Calcific tendinitis.
A 6-year-old female Siamese became lame in the left hindlimb. Clinical examination revealed pain on palpation and swelling in the region of the tibiotarsal joint. Radiographs of the affected limb demonstrated soft tissue swelling at the level of the tarsus, on the medial side (arrow). In addition, a linear pattern of calcification (arrows) was seen within the Achilles tendon or tendon sheath.

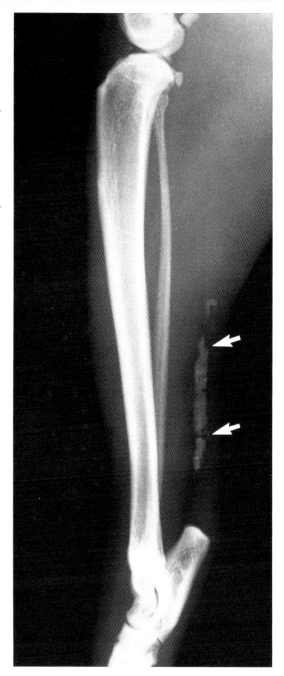

INDEX

Figure numbers are marked in bold type. Page numbers are marked in medium type.